Eat to Beat
Alzheimer's

Francie Healey

Eat to Beat Alzheimer's

Delicious Recipes and
New Research to
Prevent and Slow Dementia

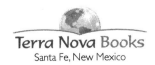

Terra Nova Books
Santa Fe, New Mexico

SPECIAL BONUS:

This may be the last book about Alzheimer's prevention you ever buy.
Owners of this book get access to the author's website and blog, with additional delicious recipes and continually updated reports on the latest Alzheimer's research: www.EatToBeatAlzheimers.com.

Library of Congress Control Number: 2015956143

Distributed by SCB Distributors, (800) 729-6423

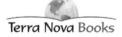

Terra Nova Books

Copyright © 2016 Francie Healey

Published by Terra Nova Books, Santa Fe, New Mexico.
www.TerraNovaBooks.com

ISBN: 978-1-938288-61-6

Contents

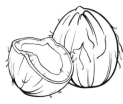

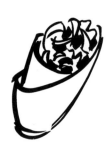

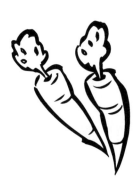

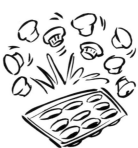

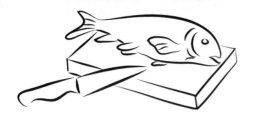

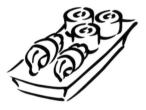

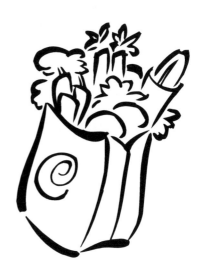

Preface

"Francie, you can write your own cookbook."
These words, spoken to me by my stepfather, John Q. Durkin, on a June day in 2012, turned my focus and life in a new direction. At the age of sixty-three, he had undergone his second surgery for cancer, and we were waiting anxiously in the hospital room for the surgeon. I had an opportunity to be alone with John, which was very unusual. I had flown in from New Mexico to New York City, not sure what I would encounter. I was completely unprepared to see my stepfather in this frail condition.

While we waited for the doctor, I felt John's fear, vulnerability, and anxiety. I had never been in this position with him before. The feeling in the room was unfamiliar to me. I had thought he was immune to fear. I became aware that it was my time to show up for John in a way that I had never imagined. It was my time to access the best of me, the parts that had been in training for this moment. It was my time to transcend our history, offer my presence, and show up to create the space of calm. It was our time.

At that moment of awareness, something shifted in the room. It felt different. It felt as though time had stopped and

These words, spoken to me by my stepfather, John Q. Durkin, on a June day in 2012, turned my focus and life in a new direction.

we could really see each other clearly. I felt the purity of the love between us. We began to have an exchange that was effortless. We were not scared—we were inspired.

In the midst of John's vulnerability and profound pain, he attuned to me and my life, my passions and my experiences. He gave his loving attention to me, and I felt seen and free. John asked about my work as a health counselor and writer.

At that point in my life, I was working too hard for too little, still too afraid to venture out on my own and trust in my own ideas of what to write, and how best to be of service to others. But the moment had come when I had to either sign away my right to have my own voice in the world of nutrition that I care about so deeply, or walk away and build something of my own. I wish I could say it was easy, but the truth is that I have struggled my whole life with having a voice. It has always been easier to let another person have the final say, or be right, or be an expert. In almost all areas of my life, I had relinquished my own opinions and perspectives again and again for the sake of keeping the peace and not rocking the boat. I had spent my life feeling that playing submissive and small would keep me safe.

I know I am not alone in this pattern, and have met many others who struggle with the same dilemma. How can we be ourselves when that requires not going along with the status quo? Whether it's the status quo of an organization we work for, a relationship we're in, or even a culture that we call home, the challenge remains the same. But there came a point in my life that highlighted this fear of really being myself and living my full potential, and it centered on my encounter with John, the stepfather who had been the world to me growing up, whose approval and love I had always worked to gain. I wanted him to see me as valuable and good, someone worth getting to know, and of whom he could be proud.

After I made the vulnerable choice to walk away from a writing job that I thought gave me professional security, I found myself in that hospital room with John, looking at the only father I have known—and at a man, beyond that, who was dealing with illness and facing the end of his life. He knew it, and I knew it. And somehow my willingness to be there with him in that way, to not deny the end but to face it, helped us both transcend the fear that could have kept us hiding behind the thin, polite veil of social graces instead of accepting the fullness of the moment and allowing the fullness of our connection to be felt and understood.

In that moment, I knew myself loved and seen in a way I never had felt before in our relationship. The few hours or so we spent together then has permanently changed the way I understand myself and how I live in the world. It completely validated my choice to walk away from a professional situation that was undermining my integrity, and to take the leap into writing this book and pursuing my own passion and enthusiasm for conscious wellness. John's deep listening, guidance, and suggestion that I write my own cookbook were the seeds for what you now hold in your hands.

As you will see, my focus on health and wellness is broad and widespread—addressing not only nutrition from a physiological perspective but also the psychological value of mindset as a critical key to how we view and value ourselves. The loving attention John showed me in that small hospital room shifted my own perspective to give my psychological health priority over the old pattern of trying to take care of others. In other words, I understood my value in a solid, foundational way, which led me to take the necessary steps to branch out on my own as a writer and health professional.

After the loss of my writing job, and my father, I encountered one more transformative experience that further propelled me into this book. Nearly a year after John's passing, I fell from the top of a fifteen-foot rock climbing wall in an accident that shattered bones and left me hospitalized. I underwent extensive surgery, had to learn to walk and use my body all over again, and still must live with ongoing pain and need for physical therapy treatments. Similar to how my encounter with John helped me recognize and love myself in a deep way, the accident forced me to stop taking care of others and open up to the help and support of my community.

For the first time in my life, I had to let go and not be the strong one. I had to allow others to cook for me, clean for

As you will see, my focus on health and wellness is broad and widespread—addressing not only nutrition from a physiological perspective but also the psychological value of mindset as a critical key to how we view and value ourselves.

me, take care of my body for me, take care of my children and my home. I was physically unable to function as I had done and was forced to slow down, rest, recover, and ultimately trust at an even deeper level that I was supported and cared for, and that even in the midst of pain and brokenness, a larger purpose was guiding my life.

Indeed, the experience of being physically unwell and incapacitated drove me to focus even more on the people and projects that are most important to me. Not only that, but my physical body in its recovery now demands more of my attention and loving care than ever before. I understand through my own experience how demanding it can be to live in a body that needs special care and how empowering it is to provide for myself the best choices possible in health, lifestyle, and diet.

Though I know in my heart that my life has been a long lesson in learning to trust myself, to be as fully authentic as I can, these three events in three years were crucial to my awakening. I believe these experiences have helped me get to the point where I could write this book and share my passion about healthy living and wellness with the world. It is my hope that in sharing this part of my story, readers will see their own lives as a guide toward their own wellness. Difficult life events can lead us to where we really want to be even if it's not visible in the moment. And my hope also is that in sharing my experiences, readers will see value in this book that goes beyond information and education to a shared dialogue on wellness—and to an awakening into the truth of who we are as a direct way to access one's own best health.

Difficult life events can lead us to where we really want to be even if it's not visible in the moment.

So, John was right in his suggestion. I did have the ability to write this book. I had worked for many years as a health counselor and researcher, educating my clients about health, nutrition, and the relationship between physical and mental health. It was time to expand my scope of work and follow John's guidance and intuition. His vision that I could make a difference has motivated me for the last three years. John's memory helped me stay committed to the completion of this project and the manifestation of his vision.

John passed away January 6, 2013. This book is inspired by him. John's spirit is infused in this work and in me.

Eat to Beat Alzheimer's

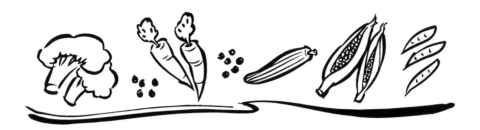

Introduction

Research tells us that people born today, or fifty years ago, to a parent with Alzheimer's disease (A.D.) are likelier to contract the disease themselves. Many of these individuals struggle with that thought every day—and, more important, with the question of how they can prevent or delay that outcome.

While there is no known cure, there is increasing evidence for the role of diet and nutrition in preventing and slowing Alzheimer's disease.

Alzheimer's, other forms of dementia, and cognitive brain decline are increasing, and are responsible for great fear in today's aging population. Additionally, in the absence of effective prevention and treatment, the forecast is a major concern to the medical and health-care communities. Roughly 5.4 million people suffer from A.D. in the U.S. alone. Nearly one in every five Medicare dollars is estimated to be spent on people with A.D. and other forms of dementia. By 2050, this is expected to be one in every three dollars. The burden on the Medicare system—and society as a whole—will be immense without changes in our approach to care.

There is increasing evidence for the role of diet and nutrition in preventing and slowing Alzheimer's disease.

This cookbook incorporates attainable prevention strategies based on knowledge from current scientific studies about how to reduce your risk of developing A.D.

This cookbook incorporates attainable prevention strategies based on knowledge from current scientific studies about how to reduce your risk of developing A.D. Shifts in the brain begin decades before the onset of symptoms, and any nutritional change you make now will benefit your brain health throughout your future. This cookbook is designed to educate readers about how to cook in a brain-protective way, so as to crowd out inflammatory foods that diminish brain health. With no known cure and limited treatment options, prevention or delay is what you have left, and how you eat is a critical part of any prevention plan. Ongoing clinical trials are gathering further information on how diet and lifestyle can help reduce the risk of Alzheimer's disease.

As we age, we become more susceptible to progressive and debilitating diseases, such as Parkinson's and Huntington's as well as Alzheimer's, which result in the degeneration and/or death of nerve cells.

Of great interest to the nutritional and aging research communities is examining the progression of cognitive disease. In addition, exciting recent studies are showing that the progression can be slowed—that is, onset of these conditions can be delayed—by following an anti-inflammatory diet and incorporating specific medicinal foods, herbs, spices, and healthy fats. The recipes in this book take advantage of these beneficial foods while providing a guide for a lifetime of eating well.

With that in mind, my vision is to help you build a connection with the healing properties of food. We live in a culture of disconnect with food. I want to empower and inspire you to change the trajectory of your health and well-being by recognizing and incorporating the medicine of food. In a prediction attributed to Thomas Edison, "The doctor of the future will give no medicine but will interest patients in the care of the human frame, in diet, and in the cause and prevention of disease."

This book is an invitation to adopt healthy, sustainable dietary changes. Food can be used as a medium to foster well-being. When we access the medicinal properties of food, it impacts our long-term health in a profound way. The earlier we invest in our health by incorporating preventive agents into our diet, the more likely it is that we can alter the course of cognitive decline. Building connections between your food and brain health builds sustainable lifestyle changes. When we choose health and reach toward our own well-being, we find our renewable resource—the inherent joy that is who we really are.

This cookbook is full of research-based nutritional information for your benefit and health. I hope that you find it educational and are empowered with the knowledge to start investigating your own individual health goals and needs. Research findings based on nutritional science are a great and positive place to start one's journey of health. However, it consists of far more than using the information. It is a journey of self-awareness first and foremost, of discovery and attunement with self that helps us really listen to our own innate feedback systems.

Use this information as a guide. In collaboration with current science, you can find a diet and lifestyle practice that honors your personal uniqueness. In addition to diet, our relationship to ourselves (and our health) holds the keys to wellness. We are not meant to become perfect beings; we are meant to profoundly care for and respect ourselves, to hear our own messages and our own guidance, and to respond with compassion, integrity, and willingness so that we can heal from what ails us.

Recipe Intentions

These recipes are delicious and nourishing for your whole body. Their purpose is to give you the knowledge and tools to take charge of your health by incorporating healing foods into your diet. The recipes promote optimal wellness, and while they are geared toward improving brain health, they are also created to be beneficial and tasty for everyone in the family. All the recipes are designed with a whole-body approach, and are rich in nutrition, flavorful, and loaded with nourishing ingredients.

All the recipes are designed with a whole-body approach, and are rich in nutrition, flavorful, and loaded with nourishing ingredients.

The B vitamins found in foods such as leafy, dark green vegetables which are incorporated in these recipes are a significant part of a brain-healthy diet and have been shown to reduce cerebral atrophy in the gray matter regions specifically vulnerable to the A.D. process.

In addition, vegetables contain phytochemicals, which, besides giving plants their flavor and color, are part of their defense system against disease; when consumed, they bring the same protective benefits—the same disease resistance —to our bodies.

A literature review published in the *Journal of Nutritional Biochemistry* reported, among other promising results on nutrition and aging, that individuals who increased their intake of vitamins and trace minerals showed a "significant improvement in all cognitive tests except long-term memory recall."

A 2011 study in the journal *Expert Review of Neurotherapeutics* stated that, "The limited epidemiological evidence available on fruit and vegetable consumption and cognition generally supports a protective role of these macronutrients against cognitive decline, dementia, and A.D."

The recipes in this book also make liberal use of healing herbs. Ongoing research in the use of specific herbs to delay and prevent cognitive decline has yielded exciting results. In particular, turmeric, ginger, and curry powder are anti-inflammatories and antioxidants, and have beneficial components for treating and preventing A.D. In addition, cinnamon has been shown to alleviate factors associated with Alzheimer's disease. The recipes here also use nourishing fats such as coconut oil and olive oil which have been found to benefit the brain.

Eating well is not about strictly following rules. It is about learning and listening. Research in the field of nutrition and health is ongoing. This exciting growth in knowledge is happening worldwide. We can educate ourselves about our own conditions and our own unique goals. And we can listen—deeply listen to our own bodies, feelings, and intuitions. We can become quiet, letting go of what we think we knew about who we are, and can listen again to the voice inside

Ongoing research in the use of specific herbs to delay and prevent cognitive decline has yielded exciting results.

that tells of a life in harmony with growth, healing, and the evolution of our own being.

Sustainability

One of this book's main goals is inspiring readers to start thinking more sustainably about what we are eating. Our nutrition does have the power to sustain our energy and health. In addition, as we discuss sustainability, consider as well the mindset of flexibility. There is no perfection or ideal we are seeking to achieve. What is attainable is a deeper understanding of yourself based on being present, deep listening, and self-reflection, as well as empowering yourself to make well-informed choices for your own health.

That deeper understanding also comes from experiencing contrasts, such as those moments when we choose something unfamiliar, or new, or ignore our own needs. Sometimes this happens for the best of reasons. It happens to everyone, and—it is important to note—is a huge part of the learning process. If we never try things outside our "normal" guidelines, we never learn where our "edges" are. And knowing that is a valuable awareness to have. It provides a working set of boundaries that can build self-trust and self-compassion—both essential for sustaining long-term healthy-living choices. The key to conscious wellness is learning, exploring, and responding to oneself over and over again, knowing when to respect our boundaries and when to push them.

Living life by following a specific diet in a rigid, rule-following way is not sustainable. Ongoing self-exploration is. Build a relationship with yourself that will keep you at the forefront of your own health journey. Be the student of your needs, and the expert on your own intuition. This is the kind of alignment that is at the very core of flexible, fluid, and loving sustainable care.

The key to conscious wellness is learning, exploring, and responding to oneself over and over again, knowing when to respect our boundaries and when to push them.

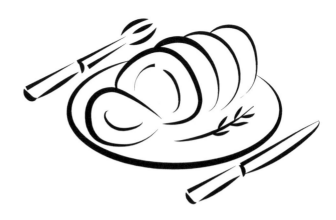

How Dementia Affects Us

As we get older, we become more susceptible to neuro-degenerative diseases connected to the aging process, with memory loss and brain atrophy as particular features. An increased risk of brain atrophy is found often in elderly persons with mild cognitive impairment. To alleviate the health-care costs and increase the quality of living for the aging population, it is crucial to explore ways of slowing or preventing the detrimental effects of cognitive decline.

According to the Alzheimer's Association—the world's leading voluntary health organization focused on Alzheimer's care, treatment, and research—dementia is a general term for a decline in mental ability severe enough to interfere with daily life. This might involve thinking, memory, learning skills, or any combination of them. Dementia is not a specific disease. It is an overall term describing a wide range of symptoms associated with a decline in memory or other thinking skills that is severe enough to reduce a person's ability to perform everyday activities.

Dementia is not a specific disease. It is an overall term describing a wide range of symptoms associated with a decline in memory or other thinking skills that is severe enough to reduce a person's ability to perform everyday activities.

The most common type of dementia is A.D., accounting for 60 to 80 percent of the cases. Vascular dementia, which usually occurs after a stroke, is the second most common type, accounting for approximately 10 percent; other forms include Lewy body and mixed dementia.

A.D. is a progressive neurodegenerative disease in that the symptoms gradually worsen over a number of years. Initially, it appears in a transitional phase known as mild cognitive impairment, which is characterized by selective memory loss. Half of all patients with mild cognitive impairment will go on to develop Alzheimer's. As the Alzheimer's Association defines it, mild cognitive impairment causes changes serious enough to be noticed by the individuals experiencing them or by other people but not severe enough to interfere with daily life or independent functioning. Those with late-stage Alzheimer's lose the ability to engage in conversation or respond to their environment.

A.D. is not considered a normal part of aging, although the greatest known risk factor is increasing age, and most people with Alzheimer's are 65 or older. But Alzheimer's is not just a disease of old age. Up to 5 percent of those with the disease have early onset Alzheimer's, which often appears when people are in their forties or fifties.

According to the World Health Organization's Dementia Fact Sheet, as of March 2015, 47.5 million people worldwide had dementia, with 7.7 million new cases every year.

The World Alzheimer Report 2015—compiled by Alzheimer Disease International, the umbrella organization of more than eighty Alzheimer's associations around the world—estimated the total worldwide cost of dementia at $818 billion. The report, titled The Global Impact of Dementia, an Analysis of Prevalence, Incidence, Cost, and Trends, also estimated that by 2018, dementia will become a trillion-dollar disease, rising to $2 trillion by 2030. The Alzheimer's Association reports that in 2015, Alzheimer's and other forms of dementia cost the United States $226 billion, estimated to rise to $1.1 trillion by 2050. "If global dementia care were a country, it would be the eighteenth largest economy in the world, exceeding the market values of companies such as Apple and Google," the association said.

A.D. is a progressive neuro-degenerative disease in that the symptoms gradually worsen over a number of years.

According to the U.S. Centers for Disease Control (CDC):

- The number of people with the A.D. doubles every five years beyond age 65; and

- Alzheimer's is the sixth leading cause of death in the United States as well as the fifth leading cause among people ages 65 to 85.

Because of the population's aging, the estimated 5 million Americans 65 years or older who had Alzheimer's disease in 2013 is projected to rise to 14 million by 2050, a nearly three-fold increase .

Deaths resulting from Alzheimer's disease are increasing, unlike those for heart disease and cancer which are on the decline. The 71 percent rise in deaths attributed to A.D. from 2000 to 2013, while those due to heart disease dropped 14 percent, led Congress to approve the National Alzheimer's Project Act to increase the funding for research, prevention, and treatment. And actually, the proportion of older people who die from Alzheimer's is believed to be considerably higher, since dementia has been shown to be under-reported on death certificates.

It is far preferable to prevent the disease as early as possible, even before the mild cognitive impairment stage begins. Diet and lifestyle offer new opportunities to achieve this prevention, as well as to improve the management of dementia that has already begun. This book explores exciting nutritional interventions shown by research to have beneficial effects in lowering oxidative stress and inflammation, with a resulting profound impact on the future of your brain's health.

Diet and lifestyle offer new opportunities to achieve this prevention, as well as to improve the management of dementia that has already begun.

Nutrition and Brain Health

The brain is the most metabolically active organ in the body. Though it accounts for approximately 2 percent of our body weight, it uses 20 percent of the body's energy. It requires a constant source of fuel to maintain its functioning.

Exciting new research is demonstrating the profound impact of food on brain health. Using that information, this book is intended to educate and inspire you to invest in the nourishment of your brain.

Until recently, the connection between nutrition and brain health was widely overlooked. But now exciting new research is demonstrating the profound impact of food on brain health. Using that information, this book is intended to educate and inspire you to invest in the nourishment of your brain.

The book's cornerstone is the role of diet and nutrition in maintaining brain health. Scientists are increasingly examining the role of foods at both ends of the spectrum: those that offer brain-boosting benefits and those that impair cognition. What they have learned gives us an opportunity to return to the ancient wisdom of food, and to incorporate its healing properties in our lives. The food we eat can either nourish or deplete the brain. Which do you want to choose?

The cost of making food selections over time that deplete the brain is profound. Most of the chronic diseases in our society—such as diabetes, high blood pressure, and cognitive impairment—are either caused or worsened by nutrition patterns over time. By investing in the brain's health, we can change our relationship with our bodies in a significant way. It is possible to experience more energy, vitality, focus, enhanced cognition, and mood stabilization by incorporating healing foods into our diets. The key is making sustainable changes in your eating habits to maximize the benefits of optimal wellness.

How to Begin Eating Well for Brain Health

As we become more disconnected from our food—such as by eating more "convenience" foods because we see our lives as too full to do otherwise, or by mindlessly picking up "healthy" food in a box—we unknowingly increase the inflammation in our bodies.

As you embark on the road to strengthening the health of your brain, I recommend starting with whole foods and crowding out processed foods. "Whole foods" are those that are unprocessed and unrefined (or processed and refined as little as possible). They typically do not contain added salt, carbohydrates, or fats. These foods remain simple and elegant with their whole vitality intact.

Foods that are refined and processed lose their wholeness and essential nutrients. Commercial processing of the food changes it from its natural state and often adds harmful ingredients as well, including sugar, artificial flavors, colorants, texturants, and preservatives. Processed foods offer us more convenience, but that comes at a high cost to our health. According to the World Health Organization, processed foods are a primary contributor to the spike in obesity levels and chronic disease around the world.

Frequent consumption of sugar and an excess of processed foods—an amount that differs for each body—has a negative effect on brain function, which contributes to declining memory and cognitive impairment. Sugar's harmful effect was shown by researchers at UCLA who discovered in a 2012 study on rats that a diet high in fructose, or fruit sugar, hinders learning and memory by slowing down the brain.

The rats who consumed excessive fructose were found to have impaired communication among their brain cells. A heavy sugar intake, the researchers found, caused the rats to develop resistance to insulin, a hormone that regulates the function of brain cells and controls blood sugar levels. In doing its work, insulin supports the synaptic connections among brain cells, aiding the part of the brain responsible for memory. The UCLA study demonstrated that lowering of insulin levels in the brain because of excess sugar consumption can impair cognitive functioning.

The recipes in this book limit processed food and sugar, which is a simple carbohydrate. All simple carbohydrates are made of just one or two sugar molecules. They are the quickest source of energy, as they are digested very rapidly. But though moderate use is fine, too much sugar over time causes surges of insulin release which lead to inflammation in the brain that can promote the development and worsening of A.D.

Sugars such as fructose, glucose, and corn syrup are found in high concentrations in processed foods. Although

The recipes in this book limit processed food and sugar.

the World Health Organization recommends that only 5 percent of our daily caloric intake come from sugar, government data shows that the typical American diet from 2005 to 2010 received approximately 13 percent of its calories from sugar.

The Impact of Excess Sugar on the Brain

A study funded by the National Institute on Aging and published in the *Journal of Alzheimer's Disease* tracked 1,230 people ages 70 to 89 who provided information on what they ate during the previous year. During that time, the participants' cognitive function was evaluated by an expert panel. Approximately 940 participants who showed no signs of impairment were asked to return for follow-up evaluations. About four years into the study, 200 of the 940 were starting to show signs of mild cognitive impairment that were greater than normal age-related changes. Participants with the highest sugar intake were 1.5 times likelier to experience mild cognitive impairment than those with the lowest levels.

Participants [in the study] with the highest sugar intake were 1.5 times likelier to experience mild cognitive impairment than those with the lowest levels.

Looking at possible reasons for this, Dr. Rosebud Roberts, a Mayo Clinic epidemiologist and lead author of the study, said: "Sugar fuels the brain, so moderate intake is good; however, high levels of sugar may actually prevent the brain from using the sugar—similar to what we see with Type 2 diabetes."

Carbohydrates are necessary for our bodies as a source of glucose which we use as fuel. They can be either complex or simple carbohydrates. Complex carbohydrates, which offer essential nutrients, contain some sugar (like fructose in fruit), starch (think of a potato), and fiber (the indigestible fibers in all natural fruits and vegetables). Simple carbohydrates are sugar without the starch and fiber (such as cane sugar, table sugar, brown sugar, corn syrup, soft drinks, fruit drinks, candy, and jam). Packaged baked goods, white bread, white rice, and white flour are all also considered simple carbohydrates because their sugar content is very high and their nutrient content (starches and fibers) is typically low.

These carbs are rapidly metabolized by the body and cause a significant rise in blood sugar levels.

In contrast, complex carbohydrates, such as green leafy vegetables, quinoa, millet, amaranth, brown rice, beans, and nuts are not as easily metabolized by the body and elevate insulin levels more gradually. Complex carbohydrates have a more-robust nutrient spectrum and do not cause the spike in blood sugar that simple carbohydrates do. This is preferable because insulin spikes and crashes are unsustainable for the body. Over time, spikes in insulin, which affects how the brain metabolizes glucose, also cause inflammation in the brain. When insulin spikes (from chronic high sugar diets) continue, glucose metabolism is disrupted, which impairs the functioning of our brain cells.

Over time, spikes in insulin, which affects how the brain metabolizes glucose, also cause inflammation in the brain.

When blood glucose (blood sugar) increases after we eat carbohydrates, the pancreas releases the hormone insulin, which helps bring the glucose to the body's cells. Too much or too little glucose in the blood can be dangerous. This is referred to as hyperglycemia or hypoglycemia, respectively. Our cells can hold only a maximum amount of glucose, so any extra returns to the liver for processing into glycogen. Glycogen is essentially stored fuel and resides in the liver and muscle tissues. Because there is also a maximum level of glycogen that can be stored there, any excess is converted into triglycerides (fat) for longer-term storage and placed in fat storage cells, or adipocytes. In the other type of imbalance that occurs, too little glucose in the system can lead to a shortage of energy and an inability to perform normal functions.

While glucose from carbohydrates is an essential nutrient for health, our bodies work very hard to maintain a delicate balance of blood sugar so that we are operating optimally. Eating high amounts of sugars and more carbohydrates than necessary places undue stress on the system to first process and use the glucose, then storing it as fat if there is too much. Continually flooding the system with sugars stresses the liver and the pancreas to convert it into glucose and transport that glucose to the cells. Our cells also become stressed and risk reducing their sensitivity to insulin, which can lead to insulin resistance, akin to a diabetic state. Moreover, a diet that is high in carbohydrates, especially refined carbohydrates and sugar, put an overall toxic burden in the body by creating an oversupply of oxidants.

Oxidants, also referred to as free radicals, are a natural byproduct of the metabolic process at the cellular level. They have roles in cell communication and cell homeostasis, and also signal inflammation. Free radicals can damage cells if they are not controlled by antioxidants. When there are more free radicals than can be managed, oxidative stress occurs, resulting in inflammation and damage to cells and tissues.

Oxidative stress and inflammation have direct effects on our brain health. But lowering the intake of sugars and highly refined, simple carbohydrates can decrease this stress and inflammation in the body and brain. Additionally, it is beneficial to incorporate more antioxidant foods in the diet (such as olive oil, blueberries, whole fruits, and vegetables).

Studies have shown that over time, sugars and high glycemic loads contribute to increases in blood sugar, which has a negative impact on your risk of developing dementia.

Studies have shown that over time, sugars and high glycemic loads contribute to increases in blood sugar, and the brain inflammation this can lead to raises the risk of developing dementia, particularly Alzheimer's. Post-mortem examinations of Alzheimer's patients show consistent brain inflammation. Because the incidence of A.D. has been reported to increase with insulin resistance—the body's reduced level of response to insulin—Alzheimer's has been referred to as Type 3 diabetes.

The glycemic index (G.I). is a measure that tracks how much and how fast blood sugar increases after consumption of carbohydrate-containing foods. The index ranks carbohydrates on a scale from 0–100. Low glycemic carbohydrates include green peas, green beans, onions, raw carrots, broccoli, cauliflower, nuts, and seeds. High glycemic carbohydrates include white flours in bagels, baguettes, bread, and pasta, pretzels, rice cakes, white rice, white potatoes, and pizza. High G.I. foods raise blood glucose more than foods with a medium or low G.I. Studies have found low-G.I. diets to be correlated with a decreased risk of cardiovascular disease, Type 2 diabetes, metabolic syndrome, and other conditions linked to inflammation.

Glycemic load measures the relative quality and quantity of carbohydrates in the diet. It applies the glycemic index to serving size and provides a clearer guide for eating to modulate blood sugar levels. Eating foods with a lower G.I. matters, but so does the amount of carbohydrates we are consuming per serving. Glycemic load takes into account a larger context for the diet by applying G.I. to portion size. In general, avoiding simple carbohydrates and focusing a person's diet on quality proteins, fats, fiber, whole fruits, and vegetables will help avoid drastic and chronic increases in blood sugar, which will decrease inflammation and promote overall health.

What is Inflammation, and How Does It Affect Our Brain Health?

Interestingly enough, the brain has no pain receptors, so it can feel no pain. When other parts of the body experience inflammation, which is our immune system's response to acute wounds or infection, they alert us with pain and discomfort—but not the brain. Instead of pain, we can recognize inflammation in the brain by its effects on functioning. Symptoms of brain inflammation are widespread, depending on where the inflammation occurs. Typical symptoms include fatigue, depression, and anxiety. In fact, depression is often an initial symptom of many neurodegenerative disorders. When the inflammation is chronic—as is common in A.D. and many other neurodegenerative disorders—the immune system has no rest; it is in a war without end. But when we change our diets to stop fueling that inflammation, we literally give our bodies a chance to experience peace, restoration, and regeneration.

When the inflammation is chronic —as is common in A.D. and many other neurodegenerative disorders—the immune system has no rest; it is in a war without end.

Chronic inflammation and chronic disease result from a variety of factors. Genetics play a role, as well as lifestyle habits, chronic stress, environmental exposure to toxins and infections, and diet. While we cannot control factors like genetics or some environmental exposure, we can make diet and lifestyle changes to address and bring down inflammation. The approach of this cookbook is to educate you on how diet choices can reduce inflammation in the brain and other parts of the body. This includes a scientific understanding of how certain foods—such as sugar and other carbohydrates, essential fatty acids, and anti-inflammatory spices—can affect our health.

The federal government's Neuroinflammation Working Group reports that, "It is indisputable that neuroinflammation occurs in the A.D. cortex." There is a clear association between inflammation of the brain and A.D. According to a study published in the journal *Neurology of Aging* in 2000, "By better understanding A.D. inflammatory and immunoregulatory processes, it should be possible to develop anti-inflammatory approaches that may not cure but will likely help slow the progression or delay the onset of this devastating disorder."

Atrophy, or shrinkage, of the brain is a normal part of aging. It occurs in cognitively healthy older adults. The rate of atrophy in Alzheimer's patients is much faster than normal, and those with mild cognitive impairment show an intermediate rate of atrophy. Inflammation and oxidative stress (the overabundance of free radicals in the body) play important roles in brain aging.

Markers of inflammation and cellular damage that naturally increase during normal brain aging help scientists track the body's level of inflammation. These are often proteins whose concentrations can be measured in blood plasma. During aging, the increase in inflammation interferes with normal glucose metabolism (how the brain uses glucose for fuel). The resulting failure in energy conversion depletes the brain cells, eventually causing them to deteriorate and die, which in turn increases the risk of developing dementia as we age. Consider the fact that highly inflammatory diets and lifestyle habits can accelerate this natural aging process, causing premature cognitive decline and disease.

It is only in recent years that we have learned of the profound impact of diet on brain health. Though the foods we eat have a powerful effect on our health in general, this is particularly so for inflammation, with highly processed and refined foods like packaged baked goods being the main dietary contributors to chronic inflammation.

> *By better understanding A.D. inflammatory and immunoregulatory processes, it should be possible to develop anti-inflammatory approaches that may not cure but will likely help slow the progression or delay the onset of this devastating disorder.*

In addition, the nightshade family of plants (Solanaceae) has been reported to contribute to inflammation, particularly in people who are sensitive to them or have other inflammatory conditions such as arthritis. A study published in the Journal of the International Academy of Preventive Medicine found significant improvement in over 70 percent of arthritic patients after solanine-containing foods were eliminated from their diets. Nightshades include potatoes (but not sweet potatoes or yams), tomatoes, peppers (not black pepper), eggplant, paprika, and tobacco. These plants contain alkaloid chemicals that can inhibit the functioning of some of the enzymes essential for almost all metabolic processes.

Although most of the book's recipes contain ingredients that are designed to reduce inflammation while avoiding foods known to increase it, there are a few exceptions. For example, I have included some ingredients from the nightshade family of plants despite their possible effects mentioned above. This means that, rather than strictly avoiding nightshades, it is important to pay attention to your own body's signals to identify if you are one of those individuals who have sensitivity to this plant family.

Although most of the book's recipes contain ingredients that are designed to reduce inflammation while avoiding foods known to increase it, there are a few exceptions.

One method is to eliminate all nightshades from your diet for at least eight weeks, then reintroduce them one at a time while noting potential symptoms of sensitivity. These can include digestive disturbance (including changes in bowel habits), joint pain or muscle aches, skin disruptions (such as eczema or acne), fatigue, and mood or cognitive changes (such as depression, anxiety, confusion, lack of mental alertness or focus). Blood tests can identify food sensitivities as well and may be a route to discuss with your doctor. If you find no negative reactions to the nightshade family, they can be a nutrient-dense variety of foods to include in your diet in moderation. Tomatoes, for example, are a member of the nightshade family that provides an excellent source of lycopene which has strong antioxidant properties important for bringing down oxidative stress.

Several studies indicate that diets rich in antioxidants and anti-inflammatory foods are beneficial for brain health and can protect the brain from oxidative and inflammatory damage. Phytochemicals, or phytonutrients, are biologically active compounds found in edible plants. This is a broad term that encompasses many different properties. Phytochemicals, such as the antioxidant flavonoids, increase our resistance to disease by providing a number of benefits.

Since we now know that many diseases are caused by inflammation, it serves us to make use of the anti-inflammatory agents that are available in nature. This conduit for change is where our power lies. By incorporating into our diet food-source phytochemicals, or phytonutrients—compounds from plants that increase our resistance to disease—we can alter the course of our brain health.

Since we now know that many diseases are caused by inflammation, it serves us to make use of the anti-inflammatory agents that are available in nature.

Nourishing Fats for the Brain

I am amazed by how many people are afraid of fat. Being "fat phobic" in this way is a product of the fat-free craze of the 1980s with its collective perception that fat was bad and made you gain weight. After being caught up in that mindset myself while in college, I spent years getting back on track with my intuition by eating whole, unrefined foods.

Back in the early '80s, no distinction was made between good fat and bad fat, and food manufacturers used extraordinary measures to create alternatives to fats—cheap substances created by hydrogenation to replace healthy butter and oils.

I remember when I was young eating margarine, a yellowish substance in a plastic container, and being told that it was healthier than butter. I didn't understand why butter was bad and why we were replacing it with something made with so many ingredients to mimic the taste of butter. How could something with a dozen additives be healthier than butter with cream and salt? Because of the old viewpoint that all fat was bad, margarine was promoted as a healthy alternative. In addition to the standard American diet's increase in hydrogenated oils—a toxic trans fat that increases inflammation—sugar was added to many "fat-free" foods to improve their taste.

Meanwhile, the CDC reports increasing diagnoses in the adult population of Type 2 diabetes, which is the leading cause of heart disease, stroke, and other chronic illness. Diabetes is an inflammatory condition. It is the result of an out-of-balance immune system and autoimmunity towards the pancreas.

Consider then what the effects are of long-term consumption of highly processed foods which trigger low-grade chronic inflammation, ultimately the leading contributor to chronic illness. Current findings make clear that a simple technique for making smart and healthful food choices is to eat whole foods (e.g., fruits, vegetables, and nuts) and foods that have been changed as little as possible from their original form. Always read the labels on packaged goods to learn about what you plan to ingest. By making simple choices to avoid food additives and complex ingredients (such as preservatives, sugars, flavorings, etc.) and choosing whole foods instead, you can make a big difference in bringing down inflammation in the body and reducing the risk of chronic illness.

Current findings make clear that a simple technique for making smart and healthful food choices is to eat whole foods

Fats are an essential nutrient. There are four types: saturated fat, monounsaturated fat, polyunsaturated fat, and trans fat.

- Saturated fats come from animals and are often solid at room temperature, such as butter, cream, lard, and tallow (beef fat) and also some plant fats like coconut oil and palm oil (which different from palm kernel oil). Historically, we have been advised to avoid saturated fats for reasons of heart health, but new understanding has shown that they can actually have health benefits.

- Unsaturated fats (monounsaturated and polyunsaturated) are liquid at room temperature. Chemically, unsaturated fats are missing one or more hydrogen pairs, which makes them less solid and dense than saturated fats. Monounsaturated fats are only missing one pair of hydrogens, so they are closest to saturated fats and thus easier for us to digest. Unsaturated fats include a large range of oils, nuts, and seeds, some of which contain the essential fatty acids Omega-3 and Omega-6.

Fatty acids are the building blocks of fats in the same way amino acids are the building blocks of proteins. Omega-3 and Omega-6 are called "essential" fatty acids because they are nutrients the body needs that we must get from our diet. But just consuming them is not enough: It is important that this be done in the right Omega-6:Omega-3 ratio—5:1 at most. But unfortunately, this often does not happen since the typical American diet is high in Omega-6 fats such as corn oil and sunflower oil because they are common in processed and highly refined foods.

Most Americans consume at least twenty-five times more Omega-6 than Omega-3, since there are limited natural food sources of Omega 3-fats.

• Trans fats, or trans-unsaturated fatty acids, are to be avoided and offer no health benefits, only risks. These have been manufactured to become solid at room temperature (think of margarine) and can be identified in food labels as "hydrogenated" or "partially hydrogenated" oils. The U.S. Food and Drug Administration banned them in 2015, giving companies three years to remove trans fats from their products.

"Good fats" are essential to a healthy diet. Fats help the body carry, absorb, and store the important fat-soluble vitamins K, A, E, and D. We could not function without fat in our diets. Consuming all fats—except trans fats—in healthy ratios is a way to include essential nutrients in our diets.

The toll of fat phobia has been immense, particularly on the health of our brains. Our brain, the fattest organ in the body, comprised of approximately 60 percent fat, requires good fat to function well. To simplify a complex process, we eat foods for fuel, and that food is broken down into three types of fuel: glycogen (from carbohydrates), proteins, and fats. Fats are the most efficient way for the body to store energy. Consider that every functioning organ in the body needs fuel to work optimally. Because the brain is comprised mostly of fat itself, it is highly efficient at processing fats for fuel. When the brain has optimal fuel, it functions well. Without that fuel, our brain health declines, and our cognition and mental health are profoundly impacted. All body tissues are affected by loss of nutrients, and this includes the brain. New discoveries and research are constantly showing us that the brain needs fat.

Omega-3 Fatty Acids

To balance the skewed perspective on fats, we must acknowledge that there are good fats and bad fats for your body. Omega-3 and Omega-6 are the two kinds of fatty acids that the body cannot produce itself. These are called "essential fatty acids" (EFAs) because it is essential to get them from food or supplements. Both are polyunsaturated fats, which have been found in studies to protect against Type 2 diabetes, Alzheimer's disease, and age-related brain decline.

To balance the skewed perspective on fats, we must acknowledge that there are good fats and bad fats for your body.

EFAs are required for maintenance of optimal health. Clinical observation studies have related imbalances in dietary intake of fatty acids (think about that optimal ratio of Omega-6 to Omega-3 being 5:1 or less) to impaired brain performance and diseases. EFAs, particularly the Omega-3 fatty acids, are involved in the synthesis and function of brain neurotransmitters. Neurotransmitters support communication between neurons in the brain, which is the basis for all brain functioning.

Omega-3 fats are one of the most talked-about components of a healthy brain diet. DHA and EPA (docosahexaenoic acid and eicosapentaenoic acid, respectively, the brain-activating forms of Omega-3 fats) have been shown to reduce depressive symptoms in individuals with age-related cognitive decline.

DHA, the principle Omega-3 fatty acid forming brain and heart tissue, plays a significant role in nerve function. Decreases in DHA are associated with cognitive decline in both healthy elderly patients and those with Alzheimer's. And epidemiologic studies show a beneficial role for DHA in preventing or halting the initial progression of A.D.

Omega-3 fats are also vital to cell wall and nerve cell integrity. Since there are limited natural food sources with substantial amounts of Omega-3 fats, getting enough of them in your diet can be challenging. Several studies have found that consumption of fish, the primary dietary source of Omega-3 fats, is associated with a reduced risk of cognitive decline or dementia. This cookbook shows you how to incorporate food sources with the highest concentration of these beneficial fats into your daily life.

The best food sources for Omega-3 EPA and DHA are wild Alaskan salmon, anchovies, sardines, mackerel, and herring. The other Omega-3, short-chain alpha-linolenic acid (ALA), can be acquired from vegetarian sources such as walnuts, chia, flax, hemp, and black currant.

Omega-6 fats are chemically unstable, meaning they can oxidize quickly and become rancid. Because oxidation contributes to many degenerative and inflammatory diseases as well as cognitive disorders, eating high levels of Omega-6 fats can increase your risk of inflammation.

Minimizing use of vegetable oils made from seeds, nuts, and beans such as soybean, corn, canola, safflower, sunflower, and peanut helps to reduce overall Omega-6 fat consumption. Omega-6 fats are also found in high concentrations in factory-farmed animals, as they are typically fed grains rather than grass.

Additionally, researchers have found that an excess of Omega-6 fats from cereals, processed foods, and especially vegetable oils and spreads increases the risk of inflammatory, neurologic, and degenerative diseases. These studies indicate strongly that limiting our intake of Omega-6 is essential to the health of our brains.

Healthy fats that your brain needs for optimal function include organically raised grass-fed meats, coconut oil, olives and olive oil, avocado, nuts, organic pastured egg yolks, and butter made from the milk of grass-fed cows.

······································

Several studies have found that consumption of fish, the primary dietary source of Omega-3 fats, is associated with a reduced risk of cognitive decline or dementia.

Coconut Oil

To add healthy fats to your diet, the recipes in this book rely heavily on coconut oil, which has been shown to have numerous beneficial effects on the aging brain. Coconut oil has received much attention in recent years, and has been touted as a miracle food with multiple benefits. But many critics also are skeptical of these reported health benefits and wary of the saturated fat content.

In trying to determine how the positive and negative claims actually balance out, I found surprisingly little research—but also some exciting studies showing coconut oil's promising impact on brain health. These were among the benefits, although further research is needed:

Chemically, saturated fats are made up of one of three fatty acid chains which differ in length: short-, medium-, and long-chain fatty acids. New research is finding exciting evidence that cognitive functioning improves in older adults with memory disorders who consume medium-chain fatty acids (MCFAs) such as those that make up coconut oil.

Compared with other fats, coconut oil (and the MCFAs present in it) is easy to digest, and it has been reported to improve the absorption of fat-soluble vitamins, minerals, and amino acids. Because MCFAs are digested quickly, they are used rapidly to produce energy rather than being stored as body fat. When consumed, many of the MCFAs in coconut oil are quickly converted into a major energy source for the brain, which increases cognitive function.

MCFAs also have been shown to be beneficial for neurologic disorders involving dysfunctions in glucose metabolism (the processing of carbohydrates and sugars for fuel). Normally, our bodies get glucose, the brain's primary and preferred energy source, from food. When no food is consumed for a while, blood glucose levels fall, and the brain needs another source of energy to function and survive. This is what good fats can provide, making glucose and fats both essential for healthy brain functioning. Diets that restrict either major fuel source (fats or carbohydrates) are not recommended unless under strict guidance from a doctor.

To add healthy fats to your diet, the recipes in this book rely heavily on coconut oil, which has been shown to have numerous beneficial effects on the aging brain.

Depriving our body of a main source of fuel has implications on the balance and health of the system. Research is still limited in this area, and it may be we have yet to discover the complexities of the brain's use of and need for different types of fuels.

In A.D., there appears to be a dramatic decrease in the brain's ability to use glucose. During the decline experienced with A.D. or other dementia, cerebral glucose metabolism appears to diminish as mitochondria (the part of our cells responsible for producing energy) become less efficient at taking in and using glucose. The brain becomes malnourished, and further nerve cell death occurs. Acting as a glucose substitute, ketones from the breakdown of MCFAs appear to offer the necessary simple fuel for mitochondria to use for energy. Neurobiological evidence indicates that ketones specifically from coconut oil can offer an effective energy base for the brain, seemingly explaining why coconut oil is getting so much attention. Research has found positive results with the use of MCFAs in A.D. patients. Case histories of Alzheimer's patients receiving coconut oil have indicated that it not only can stop the progression of the disease but also can bring about significant improvement.

For people concerned about high cholesterol, coconut oil has been considered a source of saturated fats that should be avoided. Nevertheless, let me reiterate that some types of saturated fats are good for you. Some 55 to 65 percent of the saturated fat in coconuts is not undesirable long-chain but medium-chain fatty acids, including the healthy fats that are beneficial to the body. If you have high cholesterol and are still concerned, consider substituting olive oil for medium to low cooking temperatures.

Olive Oil

Olive oil is popular in cooking today, and provides many health benefits. A growing body of evidence shows a strong connection between the consumption of extra virgin olive oil and the potential to ease the symptoms of Alzheimer's disease and age-related cognitive decline by potentially delaying the onset, and possibly preventing them altogether. For example, a recent animal study published in the *Journal of Alzheimer's Disease* found that extra virgin olive oil has beneficial effects on learning and memory problems found in aging. The type of antioxidants known as polyphenols, found in extra virgin olive oil, reverses oxidative damage in the brain, which is a leading cause of cognitive decline and other health concerns.

Oxidative damage is the result of excess free radicals, which are reactive atoms that contribute to tissue damage in the body. Free radicals form in the body through a number of processes. Environmental causes include exposure to air pollutants, industrial chemicals, daily stress, and inflammatory diets. Moreover, free radicals result from oxidation, which is a natural chemical process that happens as we interact with our environment whether through skin, lungs, or the digestive tract. When oxidation is high, for example, if we have excessive chronic exposure to environmental pollutants or consume substantial amounts of foods that produce large amounts of free radicals (trans fats, rancid nuts, seeds, and vegetable oils), we end up with more free radicals than can be neutralized chemically in the body. Oxidation is a normal occurrence, and we are equipped to deal with a small level of toxins (free radicals). However, when our toxic burden becomes too high, we are at risk for oxidative damage, or oxidative stress which has direct links to A.D., cancer, and other chronic diseases.

During the course of the body's normal functioning, these free radicals are neutralized in a process called "scavenging." One of the side effects of aging is the body's reduced capacity to effectively scavenge free radicals, which allows them to accumulate and damage cells. The negative effects of free radicals in the body are generally referred to as oxidative stress, and an increasing number of studies focus on using nutrition to combat oxidative stress. The brains of patients with A.D. are characterized by extensive oxidative stress, so any dietary potential to reduce this condition should be pursued.

....

The type of antioxidants known as polyphenols, found in extra virgin olive oil, reverses oxidative damage in the brain, which is a leading cause of cognitive decline and other health concerns.

A polyphenol is a type of chemical that acts as an antioxidant. Current research suggests that these chemicals may help protect against some common health problems and certain effects of aging by protecting cells against damage caused by free radicals. Polyphenols naturally occur in many fruits and vegetables as well as tea, red wine, and olive oil. Flavonoids are the largest group of polyphenols. A study published in 2008 in the *Journal of Agricultural and Food Chemistry* explores the relationship of the polyphenols present in berries to healthy aging. According to the study, "Consumption of diets rich in antioxidants and anti-inflammatory polyphenolics, such as those found in fruits and vegetables, may lower the risk of developing age-related neurodegenerative diseases." In lab tests, scientists have found that polyphenols can counteract the effects of aging, including oxidative stress caused by free radicals.

Brain Health Benefits of B Vitamins and Green Leafy Vegetables

The role of B vitamins, a group of chemically distinct vitamins that aid cell metabolism, in supporting brain health and preventing cognitive decline is becoming increasingly well understood.

The role of B vitamins, a group of chemically distinct vitamins that aid cell metabolism, in supporting brain health and preventing cognitive decline is becoming increasingly well understood. Each B vitamin plays a separate role in metabolism, and many health problems are caused by deficiencies in various B vitamins. (The term B complex refers to supplements or food that contain all eight B vitamins.)

B vitamins are found in many whole, unprocessed foods. Because the processing of sugar and flour leaves them with fewer B vitamins than their whole counterparts, the producers of these food products then add them back in, creating "enriched flour." Good food sources of B vitamins include green leafy vegetables and legumes.

B vitamins help to lower levels of the amino acid homocysteine in blood plasma, which a recent study by the Oxford Project to Investigate Memory and Ageing showed to be a risk factor for brain atrophy—the wasting away of brain tissue and progressive decline in function that is seen in many older adults as a result of Alzheimer's disease and cognitive decline.

However, high-dose B vitamin treatment has been shown to slow the shrinkage of brain volume, and B vitamin treatment also has been found to reduce gray matter atrophy in regions of the brain specifically vulnerable to Alzheimer's.

As an example, the Baltimore Longitudinal Study of Aging found that a total intake of folate (vitamin B9) at or above the recommended daily allowance is associated with a reduced risk of Alzheimer's disease. And the Chicago Health and Aging Project found that elderly subjects who ate close to three servings of vegetables every day slowed their cognitive decline by 40 percent.

While there is certainly room for more research, it seems clear that, among their many other benefits, the B vitamins play a role in preventing and alleviating the symptoms of cognitive decline and Alzheimer's disease.

Turmeric and Curcumin

This cookbook makes liberal use of healing spices. Turmeric, a spice of particular importance to brain health, is used worldwide but is most popular in Ayurvedic and traditional Chinese dishes and medicines.

This cookbook makes liberal use of healing spices. Turmeric, a spice of particular importance to brain health, is used worldwide.

Turmeric is native to Indonesia and southern India, where it has been used for thousands of years. It is part of the ginger family. The spice, which is derived from the plant's rhizome, has become known in the West relatively recently despite its importance in the ancient Ayurvedic tradition. Turmeric is used as a main spice of curry blends and also as a food additive and dye. Medicinally, it is used in Ayurveda to treat many ailments including liver and urinary tract disease.

Curcumin, which is present in turmeric, has been shown, like the other polyphenols in most vegetables, fruits, and spices, to have antioxidant and anti-inflammatory effects.

The Indo-U.S. Cross-National Dementia Epidemiology Study showed that the incidence of Alzheimer's disease in the Indian subcontinent is the lowest in the world and among the lowest ever reported. Studies in South India, Mumbai, and the northern state of Haryana have reported Alzheimer's rates ranging from about 1 percent in rural north India (the lowest anywhere in the world where Alzheimer's has been studied systematically) to 2.7 percent in urban Chennai, in contrast to the U.S. rate of almost 10 percent. There are a variety of explanations for this remarkable statistic, but one of the most compelling is the finding that the Indian diet—with turmeric as a primary ingredient—plays a critical role in the country's avoidance of A.D.

Curcumin is a powerful antioxidant which research has shown has a promising effect on the prevention of neurodegenerative diseases.

Curcumin is a powerful antioxidant which research has shown has a promising effect on the prevention of neurodegenerative diseases. Several studies have confirmed the positive association between curcumin and the prevention and treatment of A.D.

In the past fifteen years, curcumin has become the focus of clinical trials—many still ongoing—to test its potential use for preventing and/or treating chronic illnesses such as A.D. and cancer. Thus far, the studies have shown curcumin to reduce inflammation that could lead to disease.

One study, titled "Curcumin Reduces Amyloid Fibrillation of Prion Protein and Decreases Reactive Oxidative Stress," showed that curcumin can play a healing role in the brain through inhibition of disease-causing prion proteins as well as by rescuing cells from oxidative stress. The results highlight the strong promise that daily intake of curcumin has for preventing neurodegenerative diseases like A.D. and Parkinson's.

Studies have shown no side effects or toxicity from curcumin ingested as a seasoning or spice even at the high levels of up to 2,000 mg per day in some Indian diets, and the digestive discomfort such as mild nausea or diarrhea found from high-dosage capsules are not considered alarming.

Although curcumin taken orally has poor bioavailability—a measure of the percentage reaching the circulation unchanged—taking it together with piperine (an alkaloid found in black pepper) increases the absorption—in some studies more than doubling it. Thus, it appears from a practical standpoint that adding in pepper with your turmeric seasoning will enhance its antioxidant and anti-inflammatory properties.

And though curcumin's use in this book's recipes is geared toward preventing cognitive decline, it can, like other ingredients, benefit many of the body's systems.

A Promising Future: There Is Hope

As more people are forced to deal with A.D.'s multiple ramifications, there is a greater call for novel ways to approach its management. Creative thinking beyond the traditional type of medical care is offering hope for positive progress toward improving understanding and prevention of the disease.

Dr. Dale Bredesen, the Augustus Rose Professor of Neurology at UCLA, director of the university's Mary S. Easton Center for Alzheimer's Disease Research, and founding president of the Buck Institute for Research on Aging in Novato, California, is one of these impressive, out-of-the-box researchers. The very promising holistic therapies he has developed for A.D. patients, reported in the journal *Aging* in September 2014, show the possibility of reversing the associated memory loss through a comprehensive thirty-six-point program of lifestyle changes.

Dr. Bredesen reported on ten patients for whom he developed individualized therapeutic strategies on a case-by-case basis. The program offered a holistic approach including diet changes, supplements, exercise, meditation or yoga for stress reduction, and brain stimulation. Nine of the ten participants experienced improvement in their memories within six months. Six were able to return to work. The one subject who did not improve had been diagnosed with late-stage A.D.

Although this is a small study, and more research is needed, it is very promising to see evidence that a holistic therapy plan may indeed reverse the course of the disease.

Creative thinking beyond the traditional type of medical care is offering hope for positive progress toward improving understanding and prevention of A.D.

Getting the Most From This Book—

Meals

First, how should we define "meals" through the lens of conscious wellness? Being conscious of our wellness requires that we think more deeply about our body's needs and the quality of the nourishment we provide to meet those needs.

It has been said that "food can either be the slowest form of poison or the most powerful of medicines, but knowledge is power."

We each must consider our unique biological makeup and the specific goals we have for our own health and wellness. We must be aware of the rhythm of the day and what foods will be of service to us at which time. It can help to align with the season and one's geographic location to optimize natural harvest times. For example, fresh greens in spring can serve as a tonic after a long winter. Late summer provides fresh berries to help us store up on antioxidants for the coming winter. All of this is worthwhile to contemplate as we continually make choices about what to eat. From this perspective, we can define a meal as "a balanced combination of foods that nourishes the body in its present state by providing macro and micronutrients that optimally sustain and restore the body until the next meal." With all this in mind, I urge you to allow time for integrating this new way of thinking about your meals as you take in the information in this book and begin to explore the recipes. For now, let's discuss some practical tips for guiding those daily choices about what to eat.

In our culture, we are bombarded with images showing us ideals for breakfast, lunch, and dinner: the large stack of pancakes with syrup pouring over it for breakfast with orange juice and coffee; the overstuffed sandwich with a soda and chips for lunch; a hearty meat-focused dinner with large portions of pasta, dinner rolls, and minimal vegetable options. It is effortless to conjure these images to mind because we have been exposed to them in magazines advertisements, menus, television commercials, and billboards seemingly at every turn. It is time to break out of the trance of the standard American diet and reclaim our health by becoming conscious of every meal we eat. It is time to think beyond the sandwich and the unspoken thought that vegetables only belong as a side dish with your dinner! Don't be fooled into thinking this is too much work! On the contrary, there is great joy and relief to be experienced when we are actively tuning in to our own body and needs.

> *We can define a meal as "a balanced combination of foods that nourishes the body in its present state by providing macro and micro-nutrients that optimally sustain and restore the body until the next meal."*

Moving into conscious wellness requires a few easy skills to put us on the way to feeling healthy and vibrant again. This book supplies you with the education and awareness to achieve a new and energized relationship with the food you eat. Here are some additional action steps and perspectives to adopt that will set you up for success from morning to night.

First, a little planning goes a long way. If you invest the time to remove non-nutritive foods from your house and stock up on essentials for eating well (see Pantry Staples), you've taken a huge step toward making positive choices for the future. Putting the time in now to remove highly inflammatory choices from your cabinets only sets you up for later success. Remember that the more processed a food is, the less nutrient value it has. Letting go—in fact, throwing away—foods that have little to no nutrient value is a powerful step to take in your personalized health plan. That action alone can be transformative because in the removal of non-nutrient or anti-nutrient foods (ones that actually create problems in addition to being empty calories), you are making a strong commitment to your own wellness. Think about that moment when you find yourself hungry enough to eat the first thing you can find, only to regret later choosing the snack that leads toward inflammation and disease. Removing those negative choices puts us in a position to find new "go-to" foods and change old behaviors.

Second, this book will give you insight into key nutrients to consider when making food choices. A basic template for meal planning is the presence of three macro-nutrients: high quality protein, high quality fat (yes fat!), and complex carbohydrate.

Living in conscious wellness, we initially approach our meals by assessing whether they include these nutrients. Specifically, it is always important when one is hungry to include in any snack or meal a high-quality protein source. Protein takes time to be broken down and digested by the body, which results in longer periods of sustained energy from food. Sugary snacks, in contrast, give us an initial burst of energy which is then followed by a severe crash, often leaving us more fa-

Remember that the more processed a food is, the less nutrient value it has. Letting go—in fact, throwing away—foods that have little to no nutrient value is a powerful step to take in your personalized health plan.

tigued and hungry than we were originally. Including protein helps keep us off the sugar-spike-and-crash roller coaster by providing quality fuel that our bodies can use efficiently.

Adding in high-quality fats, such as coconut oil or avocado, and complex carbohydrates, such as brown rice, root vegetables, or whole fruits (not juices), supports the body's ability to break down the protein and provides long-lasting energy for activity and brain function. Using the Meal Plan Suggestions in this book will give you ideas for meals that include not only these macro-nutrient pillars but also ingredients that are proven to be anti-inflammatory—that literally restore our bodies' and brains' health and high functioning.

To change old habits and make new informed, positive choices for our health, we need to think beyond old diet staples.

To change old habits and make new informed, positive choices for our health, we need to think beyond old diet staples such as the sandwich, for example. Both lunch and breakfast can easily be thought of much like dinner. In fact, leftover dinner food can make excellent breakfast and lunch meals! Consider leftover stews, soups, and other dinner meals for an easy, delicious, and nutritious breakfast! Not only will you be getting protein in your meal but having leftover dinners for breakfast also can be a great way of incorporating more vegetables, and thus more nutrients, into every meal of the day.

Salads can be expanded to include hard-boiled eggs and healthy, protein-packed grains like quinoa, so that lunch has vegetables as well as a hearty dose of protein and Omega-3 fatty acids.

Thinking ahead, planning a menu for the week, and using the recipes in this book to help provide nutrient-dense, delicious, and healing options will set you up for success as you make the dietary changes needed to bring down inflammation and prevent Alzheimer's and other chronic diseases.

Snacking

As we discussed about Meals, snacks are another opportunity to create healthy, balanced "mini-meals" to help sustain you throughout the day. Over and over again, pop media has promoted snacks of highly processed and packaged foods (think of potato, corn, and tortilla chips, and high-sugar fruit snacks and drinks) which we know to be very inflammatory. Thinking of snacks as mini-meals helps guide us back to making nourishing choices that are sustaining and healthy.

Nourishing energy bars, pumpkin quinoa muffins, and healthful smoothies can provide options for those times when you need something fast and on the go. However, this requires you to make them ahead of time as you prepare for your day or week ahead, which returns us to the essence of self-care: the importance of being prepared to meet your own nutritional needs on a day-to-day basis.

I acknowledge that snacks can be difficult to figure out. Let's take a step back and think about how we can nurture ourselves before we arrive at that moment when you are "starving" and rummaging for something—anything!—that's fast to eat. In those moments when we have waited too long to eat and need to put something in our mouths quickly, our biology takes over and we are more likely to make choices that aren't as aligned with our health goals as we'd like. Taking care of ourselves means planning ahead to avoid those moments as best we can. Moreover, realizing that even when it happens—*because it does happen*—we can still be kind to ourselves and use it as a learning opportunity.

The value in using our own choices and experiences as learning moments is that it helps us really know ourselves more deeply and listen to what our body is trying to communicate.

The value in using our own choices and experiences as learning moments is that it helps us really know ourselves more deeply and listen to what our body is trying to communicate. I understand that this can be a bumpy ride, but the more willing we are to listen to what our body is saying, rather than continuing to impose on ourselves an image of what we "think" healthy eating should look like (not snacking at all, for example), the more we will be on the road to our own health and empowerment. Planning and preparing meals and snacks ahead of time to provide yourself with healthy and delicious choices in the future is an act of self-care. We cooperate with nurturing ourselves in this way by choosing foods that nurture. In our choices, we collaborate with ourselves for our own well-being.

Take the time to evaluate your own needs and invest in your own well-being. Let go of the images you have adopted as "healthy eating" so you can truly attune to your own in-

Curiosity and openness are essential to receiving accurate information from ourselves and being able to respond accordingly.

dividual needs *at this time.* Our bodies, our selves, and our lives are all fluid and ever evolving. Becoming present with ourselves on a daily basis through our food choice, keeps us in a fluid and curious state. Curiosity and openness are essential to receiving accurate information from ourselves and being able to respond accordingly. Are we hungry? Or do we need to move and get outside for a while? Did that meal sit well with me? Is my digestion off? How does my body feel right now? Keep in mind that as much as our choices impact our health regarding food, so also does our ability to become present with ourselves and listen to what our bodies need *right now.* We can be a part of our own evolution, simply by showing up and being present.

Clean Out Your Pantry

Consider letting go of foods containing these top toxic ingredients:
• Monosodium glutamate (MSG)
• Aspartame
• High-fructose corn syrup (HFCS)
• Agave nectar
• Artificial food coloring
• BHA and BHT preservatives
• Sodium nitrite and sodium nitrate
• Potassium bromate
• Recombinant bovine growth hormone (rBGH)
• Refined vegetable oil
• Any packaged foods high in sugar and refined flours.

Replace them with these suggested Pantry Staples:
• **Whole sprouted grains** such as quinoa, brown rice, amaranth, millet, and oats
• **Legumes** such as lentils, chickpeas, and white and black beans
• **Nuts** such as walnuts, pecans, and almonds, and nut butters (but not peanuts or peanut butter)

• **Seeds** such as pumpkin, sunflower, pine, chia, and hemp, and seed butters
• **Spices** such as ground and fresh turmeric, cinnamon, curry powder, cloves, ground and fresh ginger, cumin, cardamom, coriander, black pepper, ground and fresh garlic, nutmeg, and oregano
• **Dried herbs** such as rosemary, thyme, marjoram, and sage
• **Canned fish** such as salmon, sardines, anchovies, and clams
• **Flour for baking** such as almond meal, coconut flour, and arrowroot flour
• **Sea vegetables** such as nori sheets, kelp, and wakame flakes
• **Sweeteners** such as honey, maple syrup, and blackstrap molasses
• **Cooking oils** such as whole unrefined coconut oil, extra virgin olive oil, sesame oil, and walnut oil
• **Canned goods** such as whole fat coconut milk, canned pumpkin, and chicken broth

Pantry Staples

The bottom line is this: Nourishing foods in your pantry become nourishing choices for meals.

This section will discuss the importance of not only stocking your pantry with healthy ingredients but also letting go of items that will only contribute to inflammation and chronic disease.

Making dietary changes is a big deal. Food symbolizes so much in our lives. It is something we share with friends and family; it is the organizing unit of community at most social events; it provides us with memories, for better or worse— your favorite dish that grandma makes or the food that gave you food poisoning. There comes a point, however, where one begins to understand that food is much more than a symbol; it is a literal experience for our body, down to our very cells. We are now beginning to understand more and more how the food we eat has the powerful ability to promote health—or not.

It is worth repeating that the more processed (changed from its original form) a food is, the less nutrient value it has. For the sake of simplicity, consider that if you don't recognize most of the ingredients on a food's label, chances are good that you can do without it. The idea is to let go of inflammatory products and replace them with whole, nutrient-dense options.

Setting up our pantries and cabinets to have wholesome healing choices is an act of self-care. By removing unsatisfactory choices from the cabinet, we avoid the willpower battle with ourselves in which biology inevitably wins. When we are hungry enough, food is food, and we lose the pause needed to consider a healthy choice. Removing unhealthy foods protects us from having to lose that battle, and a well-stocked pantry provides us with choices that will nourish our bodies and brains.

Investing in staples now provides you with foundational ingredients for the recipes in this cookbook. It is also a literal way of taking your health into your own hands. A well-stocked pantry gives you what you need to create nourishing, delicious, healing meals at home without having to run to the store or restaurant.

We are now beginning to understand more and more how the food we eat has the powerful ability to promote health —or not.

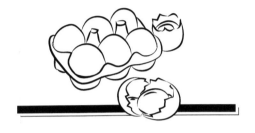

Eggs

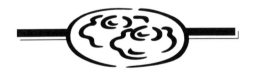

Breakfast Burrito

These inventive burritos use egg whites instead of tortillas—a great alternative for those who are trying to avoid wheat or gluten. Breakfast burritos are a hearty way to start the day, and they can be wrapped in parchment paper to carry along for a picnic. Feel free to substitute or add any vegetables you may have on hand. Bison is a bit sweeter and richer than beef, and provides a nutrient-dense, lean source of protein with as many Omega-3 fatty acids per serving as salmon. It is also rich in vitamin E and beta-carotene.

Preparation: 20 min.

Serves: 4

Ingredients

- 10 eggs
- 1 bunch green onions
- 1 cup mushrooms
- 1/4 cup cilantro
- 2 cloves garlic
- 1 avocado
- 1 lime

- 1 Tbs butter
- 1 Tbs olive oil
- 1/2 pound ground bison
- 1 tsp turmeric
- 1/2 tsp cumin
- 1/2 tsp Himalayan salt
- 1 tsp pepper

- 1/2 cup shredded cheese (optional)
- 1/2 cup sour cream (optional)

Prep
Separate eggs; put whites in one bowl and yolks in another. Chop green onions, mushrooms, and cilantro. Peel and press or finely mince garlic. Peel and dice avocado. Slice lime into wedges.

Burritos
Stirring frequently, brown buffalo in oil and butter over medium heat, crumbling meat as it cooks. Add in green onions, garlic, turmeric, and cumin. When the meat is mostly cooked, add mushrooms and continue to cook, stirring frequently, until they are soft. Stir in egg yolks and cook until set.

Meanwhile, whisk egg whites, season with salt and pepper. Pour a quarter of the mixture into a lightly oiled skillet or omelet pan. Cook very gently over low heat for about thirty seconds, then cover and cook for a minute more. Slide the egg white "tortillas" onto a plate.

Serve
Roll egg mixture into the tortillas, garnish with avocado, parsley, and a squeeze of lime. Serve with a sprinkle of cheese and a dollop of sour cream, if desired

Egg Cups

Preparation: 45 min.

Serves: 6

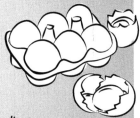

Ingredients

- 1 yellow onion
- 3 cups shiitake mushrooms
- 2 leaves kale
- 2 cloves garlic

- 1 tsp turmeric
- 1/2 tsp dried thyme
- 1/2 tsp oregano
- 1 tsp salt
- 1 tsp freshly ground pepper
- 1 Tbs olive oil
- 1 Tbs butter

- 10 eggs
- 1/2 cup parmesan cheese

- 1/4 cup parmesan

Is the morning egg routine a little boring? Try the simple act of baking your eggs in muffin tins. Not only is it a nice diversion but it also makes them portable for a picnic or snack on the go. These egg cups are packed with vitamins and minerals, featuring kale and shiitake mushrooms. Kale, which has been extensively studied for its role in cancer prevention, also has antioxidant and anti-inflammatory nutrients as well as vitamins such as A, C, and K and minerals like manganese and copper. Shiitake mushrooms have been used medicinally in Asia for 6,000 years, and are only recently becoming known in the West for their abundant benefits. They are a great non-animal source of iron, as well as pantothenic acid (vitamin B5) and selenium.

Prep
Finely chop onion, mushrooms, and kale. Peel and press or mince garlic.

Saute
In a large frying pan, saute onion, garlic, turmeric, thyme, oregano, salt, and pepper, in olive oil and butter over medium heat until onions begin to soften and spices are fragrant. Add mushrooms and kale, and continue to cook, stirring frequently, until the kale is bright green.

Bake
Distribute mushroom mixture to ten muffin tins. Crack an egg into each tin. Distribute cheese among the tins. Bake for twelve minutes at 400 degrees.

Serve
Allow to set for a few minutes before serving. Enjoy!

Mozzarella and Zucchini Frittata

Preparation: 30 min.

Serves: 4

W ith a subtle variety of flavors and textures, this lovely frittata is sure to be a hit for breakfast, brunch, or even dinner! Cremini mushrooms are high in phytonutrients. (Be sure to choose mushrooms free of discoloration, which indicates reduced phytonutrient content.) Surprisingly, cremini mushrooms benefit the immune system even more than shiitakes. Cremini are high in minerals such as copper and selenium, as well as B vitamins like B2 and pantothenic acid (B5).

Ingredients

- 1/2 red onion
- 1 zucchini
- 1/4 pound cremini mushrooms
- 7 large eggs, beaten
- 2/3 cup fresh mozzarella
- 1/2 cup fresh basil

Prep
Thinly slice red onion. Slice zucchini and mushrooms. Dice mozzarella.
Preheat oven to 350 degrees.

- 2 Tbs extra virgin olive oil
- 1/2 tsp salt

Stovetop
Saute onion, zucchini, and mushrooms in oil until soft; transfer to shallow baking dish.

- 1/4 tsp pepper
- 1 tsp turmeric

Bake
Whisk eggs, salt, pepper, and turmeric; pour over zucchini mixture.
Bake until eggs are nearly set, about three minutes. Sprinkle mozzarella and basil on top; return to oven. When eggs are done, remove from oven.

Serve
Slice and enjoy!

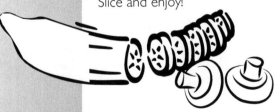

Poached Egg Bowl

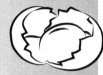

Preparation: 20 min.

Serves: 4

*T*his poached egg bowl makes a warm and gently nutritious meal. Not just for breakfast, it also can be a great lunch or light dinner. Feel free to add any leftover veggies you may have in the fridge. Quinoa and spinach are both members of the chenopod family, known for their unique carotenoids that are especially beneficial to nervous system health. Spinach is also rich in anti-inflammatory and antioxidant flavonoids. It is thought to have originated in ancient Persia, and been brought to China by the seventh century and Europe in the eleventh.

Ingredients

- Quinoa
- 2 cloves chopped garlic
- 1 chopped shallot
- 3 cups chopped spinach
- 2 carrots
- 1/2 inch ginger

- 1/2 Tbs white vinegar
- 4 eggs
- 1/2 tsp salt
- 1/4 tsp freshly ground pepper
- 2 Tbs coconut oil
- 1/4 tsp turmeric

Prep
Cook quinoa according to package directions, enough to make four servings. Peel and finely chop garlic and shallot. Chop spinach. Shred carrots. Grate ginger.

Stovetop
Heat one inch of water along with the vinegar in a shallow pan over high heat. When the water begins to simmer, lower heat to medium and gently crack eggs into the water; add salt and pepper. Continue to simmer until whites are opaque.

Saute shallot, garlic, and spices in coconut oil; add quinoa and spinach. Continue cooking until spinach is just wilted; keep warm until ready to serve.

Serve
Divide quinoa and spinach mixture into bowls; serve with an egg.

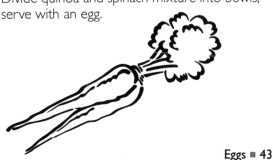

Spinach and Egg Bites

Preparation: 45 min.

Serves: 4

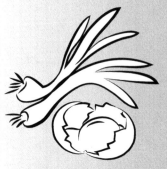

Ingredients

*M*uffin tins are not just for muffins and cupcakes! These fabulous egg bites are perfect for those busy mornings. Make a batch on the weekend or the night before, and enjoy a quick and easy breakfast. Or throw a couple in a cooler and take them with you for a nutritious mid-morning snack. Millet is thought to have originated in Ethiopia, where it has been used since prehistoric times. Although it has been in use in Africa, India, and elsewhere in Asia since ancient times and in Eastern Europe since the Middle Ages, it has only recently begun to be appreciated in Western Europe and North America. Millet is an excellent source of copper, phosphorus, manganese, and magnesium. These minerals help it to provide heart protective benefits as well as aid in repairing tissues and lowering the risk of Type 2 diabetes.

- 1 cup spinach
- 2 cups shitake mushrooms
- 1/3 cup green onions
- 1 large clove garlic

Prep
Roughly chop spinach. Chop mushrooms and green onions. Peel and press garlic.

Preheat oven to 350 degrees. Oil muffin tin, or use liners if you prefer.

- 1/2 cup uncooked millet
- 2 cups water
- 1/2 tsp salt

Stovetop
Toast millet in a medium-sized pot over medium heat, stirring occasionally. Add water and salt, cover, and increase heat to boil. Reduce heat slightly, and continue to cook until water is absorbed.

- 6 eggs
- 1 cup coconut milk
- 1/2 tsp salt
- 1/2 tsp pepper
- 1 tsp turmeric

Bake
In a medium bowl, whisk eggs, coconut milk, salt, pepper, turmeric, and garlic. Toss together with millet, spinach, mushrooms, and green onions; mix very well. Spoon into muffin cups; bake ten to twelve minutes, or until lightly firm to the touch.

- 1/2 cup shredded parmesan cheese

Serve
Sprinkle with cheese as soon as the egg bites come out of the oven; allow to cool slightly before serving.

Spinach Mushroom Frittata

Preparation: 45 min.

Serves: 4

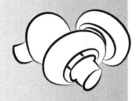

Ingredients

I like eggs and the protein they provide, but I've gotten a bit tired of them. I find this dish more interesting and enjoyable, and I like the added dimension of red potatoes. Spinach is high in antioxidants, and is a rich source of folate and vitamin C. Low folate levels are connected with poor cognitive function and dementia in the elderly. Spinach also contains a wide variety of phyto-nutrients, including flavonoids and carotenoids. Its flavor compounds have been shown to have powerful anti-inflammatory and anti-cancer properties. Depending on your sensitivity, you may want to con-sider using potatoes sparingly or leaving them out.

- 1 large shallot, chopped
- 1 Tbs cilantro or parsley
- 1½ cups shiitake or other mushrooms
- 2 cups fresh spinach
- 3–4 medium red potatoes

Prep

Finely chop shallot and cilantro or parsley. Coarsely chop mushrooms and spinach. Thinly slice potatoes.

- 8 eggs
- 1/2 cup grated parmesan cheese
- 1/2 tsp turmeric
- 1/2 tsp salt
- 6 tsp extra virgin olive oil
- 2 tsp vegetable or chicken broth

Frittata

Beat together eggs, cheese, turmeric, and salt. Set aside.

In large skillet, heat 3 tablespoons olive oil and broth over medium-low heat. Add shallot, and stir often until soft (three to five minutes). Add mushrooms and saute until tender (three to five minutes). Stir in spinach and cilantro and saute two minutes more, then add to the egg mixture.

In large skillet, heat remaining oil over medium heat, fully coating bottom of skillet. Spread red potatoes over the skillet bottom in one or two thin layers, and cook five minutes over medium heat. Pour egg and vegetable mixture over potatoes; turn heat down to low-medium, and cover. Cook about twenty minutes, periodically checking to see if eggs are firm.

Serve

When done, run rubber spatula around edge of frittata, cut in wedges, and serve.

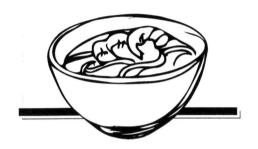

Soups and Stews

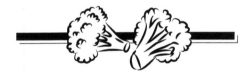

Black Bean and Sweet Potato Soup

Preparation: 1 hour

Serves: 4

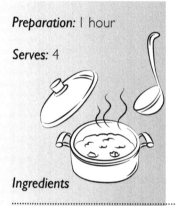

Ingredients

- 4 cups black beans
- 1/2 cup shallot
- 2 cloves garlic
- 2 large sweet potatoes
- 1 cup red cabbage
- 1 lime

- 1 Tbs coconut oil
- 1 Tbs pumpkin seeds
- 1 quart chicken or vegetable broth
- 2 cups water
- 1 tsp turmeric
- 2 tsp cumin
- 1 Tbs chili powder
- 1 tsp ground coriander
- 1 tsp Himalayan salt
- 1/2 tsp black pepper

- 1 avocado
- ½ cup cilantro

The natural sweetness of sweet potatoes, along with the protein of black beans, gives this hearty soup a satisfying heft that will sustain you between meals. The soup is loaded with vitamins and minerals as well as antioxidants and anti-inflammatories. And the cabbage also is prized for its cholesterol-lowering properties. Red cabbage offers additional nutritional benefits, including a high amount of protective phytonutrients. Enjoy this soup any time of year, and take it with you in a thermos for a burst of energy and protein during the day.

Prep

If you're using dried beans, soak half a pound overnight. Otherwise, drain and rinse two cans of beans. Peel and chop the shallot, garlic, and sweet potatoes. Chop the cabbage. Juice the lime.

Soup

In a large soup pot, heat the coconut oil over medium heat. Add in the shallot, garlic, and pumpkin seeds, and cook until tender, stirring frequently. Stir in sweet potato. Cook for five minutes. Add in broth, water, lime juice, black beans, and red cabbage. Stir well. Add the turmeric, cumin, chili powder, and coriander. Stir. Bring to a boil, then reduce heat and simmer on medium-low heat until sweet potatoes are soft, about thirty minutes.

Remove 2 cups of soup; blend with a countertop or immersion blender. Return to soup pot, stir in salt and pepper.

Serve

Peel and cube avocado, chop cilantro. Ladle soup into bowls, and sprinkle with avocado cubes and cilantro.

Broccoli and Almond Soup

Preparation: 1 hour

Serves: 4

Ingredients

- 1/2 cup slivered almonds
- 1 medium yellow onion
- 3 ribs celery
- 2 Tbs fresh parsley
- 2 cloves garlic
- 2 heads broccoli

- 1 Tbs olive oil
- 1 Tbs tamari
- 1 Tbs fresh thyme
- 1 Tbs fresh marjoram
- 1 tsp Himalayan salt
- 1 tsp black pepper
- 2 cups chicken stock
- 3 Tbs almond butter
- 1 can coconut milk

This is a delicious, creamy soup that benefits the whole body. Broccoli is a member of the cruciferous vegetable family, and has many benefits for all the body's systems. Besides its anti-inflammatory and other benefits for cognitive support, broccoli enhances detoxification, has antioxidant benefit, and also supports digestion, cancer prevention, and the cardiovascular system. Almonds reduce risk of heart disease, lower cholesterol, and protect against diabetes and cardiovascular disease.

Prep
Toast almonds in a dry skillet over medium heat; set aside. Chop onions, celery, and parsley. Peel and press or finely chop garlic. Chop broccoli; peel and chop stems as well.

Soup
In a dutch oven or soup pot, saute onion, garlic, tamari, thyme, marjoram, salt, and pepper in olive oil over medium heat until onions are soft. Add broccoli and celery, and continue to cook, stirring frequently, for five to seven minutes.

Add stock and almond butter, increase heat, and bring to a boil. Reduce heat and simmer until broccoli is nearly done, being careful not to overcook. Remove from heat; allow to cool slightly.

Using an immersion or countertop blender, puree the soup and stir in coconut milk.

Serve
Serve soup garnished with parsley.

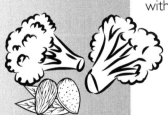

Butternut Squash Soup With Coconut and Ginger

Preparation: 40 min. active, plus 1.5 hours to bake the squash

Serves: 6

*W*inter squash plus healing herbs are a winning combination in this nourishing autumn soup. Winter squash is a wonderful source of vitamin A, which is a powerful antioxidant and has been shown to help protect against lung and mouth cancers. Enjoy this delicious, hearty soup with a bunch of friends on a crisp fall or winter day.

Ingredients

- 2 large butternut squash
- 2 Tbs pasture butter
- Himalayan salt to taste
- Fresh ground black pepper to taste
- 1 medium yellow onion, finely chopped
- 1 rib celery, diced
- 2 Tbs fresh ginger
- 1 cup chard
- 1 cup cilantro
- 1 cup coconut flakes

- 1 Tbs coconut oil
- 1 tsp turmeric
- 1 tsp curry powder
- 1/2 cup white wine
- 6 cups chicken broth
- 1 can unsweetened coconut milk
- 1 fresh thyme sprig

Prep

Preheat oven to 350 degrees. Cut squash in half lengthwise. Spread cut sides with 2 tablespoons butter; sprinkle liberally with salt and pepper. Cover cut sides with foil, and bake until tender, about an hour and a half. When cool enough to handle, scoop out flesh.

While squash is cooking, prepare remainder of ingredients. Finely chop onion. Dice celery. Peel and finely mince or grate ginger. Chop chard and cilantro. Toast coconut flakes in a dry skillet over medium heat, stirring frequently.

Soup

In a large soup pot, melt remaining butter and coconut oil over medium heat. Add onions, celery, ginger, turmeric, and curry powder; cook, stirring frequently, until onions are translucent. Add wine and cook until nearly evaporated. Add chard and cook until wilted. Mix in squash and remove from heat.

Allow to cool slightly, and puree with a countertop or immersion blender. Return to soup pot; add broth and coconut milk. Mix well. Add thyme sprig and simmer over medium-low heat for twenty minutes or until you're ready to eat! Remember to remove the thyme sprig before serving.

Serve

Sprinkle with coconut flakes and cilantro to serve.

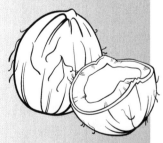

Celery Root Soup

Preparation: 40 min.

Serves: 4

Ingredients

- 1/2 cup pumpkin seeds
- 1 tsp salt
- 1 chopped medium onion
- 1 Tbs chopped fresh thyme
- 1 peeled and chopped celery root
- 2 peeled and sliced parsnips
- 1 sliced lemon

- 2 Tbs olive oil
- 1/2 tsp ground pepper
- 1 tsp turmeric
- 6 cups vegetable or chicken stock

*P*rized for its antioxidant and anti-cancer properties, celery root, or celeriac, has been cultivated since ancient times. It is a very good source of vitamin K, which limits neuronal damage in the brain, playing a valuable role in the treatment of Alzheimer's disease. Celery root also is high in dietary fiber, and adds a hearty dimension to this pretty soup, which is rich and creamy without any dairy products. It is gentle and soothing, as the pumpkin seeds add a delightful contrasting texture along with plenty of zinc and iron.

Prep
Toast pumpkin seeds in a dry skillet over medium heat. Toss with 1/2 teaspoon salt, and set aside.

Dice onion and thyme. Peel and dice celery root and parsnips. Slice lemon into wedges.

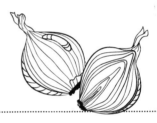

Soup
In a soup pot, saute onion in olive oil over medium heat until soft. Add remainder of salt, pepper, turmeric, thyme, celery root, parsnips, and stock. Bring to a boil, then reduce heat and simmer until vegetables are soft, about twenty minutes.

Remove from heat, let cool slightly, and puree with an immersion or countertop blender.

Serve
Serve with a squeeze of lemon juice and garnished with toasted pumpkin seeds.

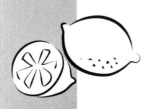

Coconut Carrot Soup

Preparation: 30 min.

Serves: 4

Coconut oil is a healthy fat, and has been shown to have numerous beneficial effects on the aging brain. It is made of medium-chain fatty acids, which have been shown to help improve cognitive functioning in older adults with memory disorders. Sweet potatoes are a good source of vitamins A and C and antioxidants. Ginger supports digestion and also has anti-inflammatory properties. This is a mild, lightly sweet soup that is popular with the whole family. I serve it over the holidays, and it is always well received.

Ingredients

- 2 Tbs coconut oil
- 1 chopped large shallot
- 2 Tbs chopped fresh ginger
- 1½ tsp curry powder
- 4 cups chicken or vegetable broth
- 5 chopped medium carrots
- 2 cups cubed sweet potatoes
- 1 can (13.5 oz.) unsweetened coconut milk
- Himalayan salt to taste
- Black pepper to taste

- 2 Tbs chopped cilantro
- 1 lime, cut into wedges

Soup

In a soup pot, heat oil over medium heat. Add shallot and a splash of broth, and saute about two minutes. Add ginger and saute another two minutes. Add curry powder, and stir until fragrant.

Add remaining broth, carrots, and sweet potatoes, and simmer on medium-high heat until vegetables are tender (about fifteen minutes). Add coconut milk, and salt and pepper to taste.

Use an immersion blender or blend in batches, making sure blender is not more than half full. Return to soup pot and reheat.

Serve

Serve piping hot in bowls garnished with cilantro and fresh lime wedges.

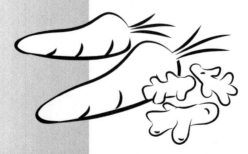

Coconut Ginger Salmon Soup

Preparation: 60 min.

Serves: 4

Shopping tip: When buying fresh salmon, ask the seller to debone it and remove the skin.

This gingery salmon soup is bright and rich—a perfect follow-up to a day outdoors. Or make it ahead of time and take some along in a thermos. Wild Alaskan salmon is an abundant source of Omega-3 fatty acids. And the healing herbs are a perfect accompaniment to salmon's Omega-3 fatty acids. This is a tasty way to prepare salmon, particularly for those who have not yet learned to appreciate salmon's many charms.

Ingredients

- 1 pound wild salmon
- 1 tsp Himalayan salt

Prep Salmon

If not already done, prep salmon by deboning it and removing the skin. Season with 1 teaspoon salt, and cut into 1-inch cubes. Refrigerate for thirty minutes while preparing the soup.

- 3 chopped shallots
- 1 Tbs butter
- 4 cups chicken stock
- 2 cans coconut milk
- 1 inch grated ginger
- 2 stalks fresh lemon grass
- 1/2 tsp red curry paste
- 1/2 tsp fish sauce
- 1 tsp Himalayan salt
- 4 oz. rice noodles
- 1 bunch chopped baby bok choy

Prep Soup

In a dutch oven or soup pot, saute shallots in 1 tablespoon butter until translucent. Add stock, coconut milk, ginger, lemon grass, curry paste, fish sauce, and salt. Bring to a boil over medium heat; cook for twenty minutes. Decrease heat to low, and simmer another five minutes.

Increase heat to medium, add salmon, and simmer for five minutes. Add rice noodles and baby bok choy, and continue simmering until rice noodles are cooked, approximately five minutes.

- 1 lime, cut into wedges
- 2 Tbs chopped cilantro

Serve

Ladle into bowls, garnish with cilantro and lime wedges.

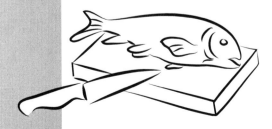

Down-to-Earth Beet Soup

Preparation: 10 min., plus 45 for roasting

Serves: 4

Ingredients

*B*eets are a naturally sweet root vegetable that is packed with vitamins and minerals. They are a good source of vitamin B and iron, as well as a source of betalains, which have been shown to provide antioxidant, anti-inflammatory, and detoxification support. B vitamins also have been shown to prevent brain atrophy. This soup is a delicious way to introduce beets into your family's repertoire. But beets' bright pigment can stain, so be careful!

- 6 large beets
- 2 finely chopped shallots
- 1/2 inch fresh ginger, grated
- Juice of two limes

Prep
To roast beets, preheat oven to 350 degrees.
   Wash beets gently to leave skin in place. Trim, leaving an inch or so of the stem and taproot. Place in a baking dish with about ½ cup water, cover, and bake until soft, about forty-five minutes. Allow to cool slightly, rub skin off, and dice.
   Peel and finely chop shallots. Grate ginger. Juice limes.

- 1 tsp ground cumin
- 1 tsp coconut oil
- 1 quart chicken or vegetable stock
- 1 15-oz. can coconut milk
- 2 Tbs cilantro

Soup
Saute shallots, cumin, and ginger in coconut oil in a large soup pot over medium heat. When shallots are soft, add beets and stock. Bring to a boil, then reduce heat and simmer five minutes. Let cool slightly, and use a blender to puree. Stir in coconut milk and lime juice.

Serve
Ladle into bowls; garnish with cilantro.

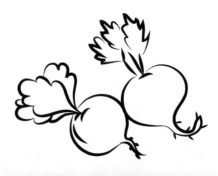

Restorative Chicken Soup

Preparation: 3 hours

Serves: 6

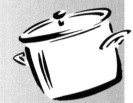

Ingredients

- 3 quarts chicken broth
- I whole chicken
- I celery root, peeled and coarsely chopped
- I coarsely chopped yellow onion
- I coarsely chopped carrot
- 6 peeled garlic cloves
- 10 whole black peppercorns
- 10 thyme sprigs

- 6 carrots
- 3 parsnips

- 1/4 cup brown mustard
- 1/2 tsp salt
- 1/2 tsp pepper
- I zucchini
- I tsp thyme

*T*his chicken soup begins with homemade broth, so it is perfect for those slow weekend mornings at home. You'll be delighted as the mouth-watering aromas fill your house throughout the day. Packed with vitamins and minerals, vegetables and healing properties, this soup truly is "good for what ails ya." Parsnips are a lovely, naturally sweet root vegetable, related to the carrot, with anti-inflammatory and antioxidant properties. They are packed with iron, manganese, and B vitamins. This soup is also very beautiful, sure to impress family and guests alike. Prepare the stock.

Prepare Soup

In a large soup pot, combine broth, chicken, celery root, onion, I coarsely chopped carrot, garlic, peppercorns, and thyme sprigs. Bring to a boil, then reduce heat and simmer until chicken is cooked, about 1½ hours. Transfer chicken to a platter, and let cool. Meanwhile, prepare the rest of the dish. Debone the chicken when cool.

Strain the broth, and return it to the pot. Discard (or compost) the veggies. Bring to a boil over high heat, skimming as necessary, until reduced to 6 cups, about fifteen minutes. Cover and keep hot.

Prepare Veggies

Peel parsnips. Dice carrots and parsnips. In a medium saucepan, bring carrots and parsnips to a boil, then reduce heat and simmer until tender. Drain and set aside. You may wish to cook the carrots and parsnips separately to preserve their individual flavors.

Combine carrots, parsnips, deboned chicken and I cup of broth in a large pot over medium-high heat; cover. Remove from heat when warm.

Serve

Stir mustard, salt, and pepper into broth. Chop zucchini into matchsticks; chop thyme.

Divide chicken and vegetables among bowls; add zucchini. Sprinkle with thyme, then ladle enough hot broth to cover.

Sunshine Stew

Preparation: 75 min.

Serves: 4

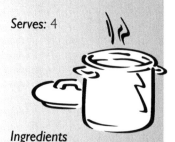

This is a brightly colored, warm, nurturing stew. Lentils are an economical way to increase your fiber, iron, and B vitamins. Pumpkin is a good vegetable source of Omega-3 fatty acids and vitamins A and C. If you are in the mood for something sweet, the natural sweetness of the pumpkin and sweet potato will fill the bill. In addition, kale is high in B vitamins, and a number of studies have shown strong evidence linking a high dietary intake of B vitamins to a lower risk of developing Alzheimer's.

Ingredients

- 1-inch piece ginger
- 3 cloves garlic
- 1 medium shallot
- 4 ounces split red lentils
- 1 small sweet potato
- 3 medium carrots
- 3 leaves kale
- 1 lime

Prep
Peel and grate ginger. Peel and press or mince garlic. Thinly slice shallot. Wash and drain lentils. Dice sweet potato. Chop carrots and kale. Slice lime into wedges.

- 2 Tbs coconut oil
- 2 tsp ground coriander
- 2 tsp ground cumin
- 1 Tbs red curry paste (optional)
- 1 Tbs turmeric
- 1 (13-oz.) can coconut milk
- 1 quart chicken stock
- 1 (15-oz.) can pumpkin puree
- black pepper, to taste
- Himalayan salt, to taste

Stew
Heat coconut oil in a heavy stockpot. Saute ginger, garlic, and shallot until shallot is translucent. Add coriander, cumin, red curry paste, and turmeric; continue to saute a few more minutes.

Add in coconut milk, chicken stock, and lentils. Increase heat, and bring to a boil for twenty minutes, stirring occasionally. Reduce heat to medium, add in sweet potato and carrots, and simmer for a further forty minutes, or until sweet potato is soft.

Just before serving, stir in kale, salt, and pepper as needed.

Serve
Ladle into bowls, and garnish with lime wedges.

Winter Squash and Bison Stew

Preparation: 10 minutes, plus 1 hour to bake

Serves: 4

Ingredients

- 1 medium winter squash
- 1 Tbs extra virgin olive oil
- 1 sweet onion
- 6 cloves garlic
- 2 celery stalks
- 2 carrots
- 3 cups broccoli
- 2 sprigs fresh rosemary
- 2 sprigs fresh thyme
- 1 bay leaf
- 1 can garbanzo beans

- 2 Tbs extra virgin olive oil
- 1 pound bison stew meat
- 1/2 tsp chile powder
- 1/2 tsp cumin
- 2 quarts beef broth
- 2 Tbs apple cider vinegar

*F*eaturing healing herbs, this lightly sweet stew will surely warm you on a crisp winter's day. Related to mint, rosemary is a small evergreen shrub prized for its aroma and flavor as well as its healing properties. Rosemary stimulates the immune system, improves digestion, and increases circulation. Native to the Mediterranean region, it is now cultivated in temperate areas throughout the world.

Prep

Preheat oven to 350 degrees.

Cut squash in half, and remove seeds. Spread oil on cut sides. Place cut side down in baking dish, and bake forty-five minutes to an hour, until squash is soft. While squash is baking, prep remainder of the ingredients.

When squash is finished, scoop out flesh and cut into bite-sized chunks.

Peel and chop onion. Finely chop garlic. Chop celery and carrots. Chop broccoli crowns, and peel and chop broccoli stems.

Place rosemary, thyme, and bay leaf in an herb bag. Rinse and drain beans.

Stovetop

Saute onions over medium heat, with extra virgin olive oil, in a large dutch oven or soup pot, until soft. Add bison and continue to cook, stirring frequently, until browned on all sides. Add garlic, celery, carrots, spices, broth, beans, and apple cider vinegar. Bring to a boil, then reduce heat. Add herb bag and simmer for ten minutes. Add broccoli and squash, and cook for a further ten minutes.

Serve

Remove herb bag and ladle stew into bowls. Enjoy!

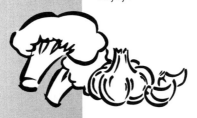

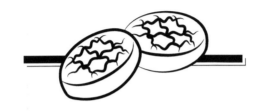

Wraps and Patties

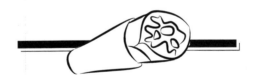

Crab Cakes

Preparation: 35 min.

Serves: 4

Ingredients

*C*rab meat is definitely a treat, as it can be rather expensive. Like all seafood, it tastes best when fresh, so it is definitely worth eating in season. However, several prepackaged alternatives exist and are readily available throughout the year. Crab has many health benefits. High in vitamin B12, it is also a complete protein and is packed with Omega-3 fatty acids. These cakes are light and tasty, and perfect on a bed of mixed greens with a squeeze of lemon.

- 1 egg, lightly beaten
- 1/2 c chopped green onions
- 2 Tbs mayonnaise
- 1 Tbs cilantro, chopped
- 16 oz crab meat
- 1 Tbs Old Bay seasoning
- 1/3 tsp turmeric
- 1/4 tsp pepper

Crab Cakes
Preheat oven to 350 degrees. Line a baking sheet with parchment paper.

Begin by preparing crab cakes. In a large bowl, combine lightly beaten egg, onions, mayonnaise, cilantro, crab meat, Old Bay seasoning, turmeric, and pepper. Mix well and form into patties. Arrange on baking sheet and sprinkle with additional Old Bay.

Bake 25 minutes, or until cooked through.

- 1/2 c extra virgin olive oil
- 3 Tbs fresh squeezed lemon juice
- 1 tsp brown mustard
- 1 clove fresh garlic, crushed
- 1 tsp raw honey

Honey Mustard Vinaigrette
While crab cakes are baking, make vinaigrette. In a small bowl, combine extra virgin olive oil, lemon juice, mustard, garlic, and honey. Whisk until well-combined, and refrigerate until ready to serve.

- 1 lemon, cut into wedges
- Fresh mixed greens of your choice

Serve
Serve on a bed of mixed greens with a squeeze of lemon and a drizzle of vinaigrette.

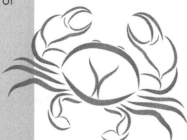

Jicama Lettuce Wraps

Preparation: 20 minutes active, plus 15 minutes to set.

Serves: 4

Ingredients

- 1/4 cup pumpkin seeds
- 1 Tbs fresh mint
- 1 bunch parsley
- 1 bunch radishes
- 1/2 pound jicama
- 2 carrots
- 1 cucumber
- 1 large avocado
- 8 kalamata olives
- 1/2 lemon

- 1/4 cup extra virgin olive oil
- 2 Tbs apple cider vinegar
- 1/2 tsp Himalayan sea salt

- 1 tsp cumin
- 1/3 cup goat cheese crumbles (optional)
- 1/2 tsp ground black pepper

- Romaine or another lettuce

*R*eminiscent of tabouli, this bright, light wrap filling is delicious as a side salad on its own or wrapped in lettuce leaves. Jicama, also known as yam bean or Mexican water chestnut, is a crisp, lightly sweet taproot vegetable. Full of phyto-nutrients, it offers fiber, antioxidants, vitamins, and minerals, and also is rich in vitamin C, B-complex vitamins, and magnesium, copper, iron, and manganese. Jicama supports the body's digestive, immune, circulatory, and many other systems.

Prep
Toast pumpkin seeds in a dry skillet over medium heat, stirring occasionally.

Finely chop mint, parsley, and radishes. Peel and finely chop jicama. Seed and dice cucumber. Peel, pit, and dice avocado. Pit and mince olives. Juice lemon.

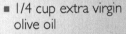

Dressing
In a small bowl, whisk together olive oil, vinegar, lemon juice, and salt.

Assemble
Combine pumpkin seeds, cumin, cheese, veggies, olives, and mint in a large bowl; mix well. Toss with dressing. Let sit fifteen minutes or more before serving.

Serve
Spoon jicama mixture into lettuce leaves and roll.

Mediterranean Turkey Patties

Preparation: 30 minutes active, plus 1 hour to set.

Serves: 4

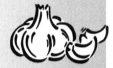

Ingredients

- 1/2 cup shallots
- 3 cloves garlic
- 2 tsp fresh thyme
- 1 Tbs fresh basil
- 3 leaves chard
- 1 lemon
- 1 Tbs mint leaves
- 1 Tbs chives
- 1 bunch green onions
- 1 cucumber

- 1 cup plain Greek yogurt
- 1/2 tsp Himalayan salt

- 1/2 tsp turmeric
- 1/2 tsp pepper
- 1/2 tsp Himalayan salt
- 1 pound ground turkey meat
- 1 Tbs hemp hearts
- 2 Tbs coconut oil

- 2 cups mixed greens

*T*he romance of northern Africa infuses these tasty patties. The rich medley of textures and flavors blends beautifully, adding interest and delight to the ground turkey, and healing herbs and spices enhance turkey's natural gifts. Turkey is rich in vitamins B3 and B6, as well selenium and phosphorus. It also provides a fair amount of Omega-3, and works to lower the Omega-6:Omega-3 ratio. Turkey is associated with a decreased risk of pancreatic cancer, and also aids in stabilizing insulin levels.

Prep

Blend in a food processor, or use a knife to finely chop shallots, garlic, thyme, basil, and chard. Set aside.

Juice enough lemon for 1 teaspoon, and zest enough lemon for ½ teaspoon. Chop mint leaves, chives, and green onions. Seed and dice cucumber.

Sauce

Toss yogurt and salt with cucumber, mint leaves, chives, and green onions. Mix well and set aside.

Patties

Mix lemon zest, turmeric, pepper, and salt with chard mixture. Fold in turkey, and mix well. Form patties and roll edges in hemp hearts. Refrigerate patties for one hour.

Fry patties in oil over medium heat, about eight minutes per side.

Serve

Serve patties over a bed of greens, drizzled with sauce.

Salmon and Sweet Potato Cakes

Preparation: 30 min.

Serves: 4

This recipe contains an abundance of protein, and salmon is a great source of Omega-3 fatty acids. Parsley is rich in antioxidant nutrients and folate, and is high in vitamin C, which acts as a co-factor for cell function and repair as well as an antioxidant. The shallots add a dimension of sweetness. My daughter, Madeleine, had three of the cakes and thought them a delicious dinner!

Ingredients

- 2 large sweet potatoes
- 1 shallot
- 1/3 cup parsley
- 1 tsp fresh rosemary
- 1 bunch green onion
- 2 lemons

- 2 6-oz. cans wild Alaskan salmon (boneless, skinless)
- 1/2 cup cornmeal
- 1/4 tsp salt
- 3 eggs
- 3 Tbs extra virgin olive oil

- 4 cups mixed baby greens

Prep
Leaving skins on, cube sweet potatoes. Finely chop shallots, parsley, rosemary, and green onions. Cut lemons into wedges.

Cakes
Boil sweet potatoes for fifteen minutes or until tender. Drain and mash in large bowl. Add drained salmon, shallot, parsley, rosemary, green onions, cornmeal, salt, and eggs. Mix well. Shape mixture into palm-sized patties (about 2 inches in diameter).

In large skillet, preferably iron, heat oil over medium-low heat. Add patties, and cook until undersides are slightly golden (about three minutes per side). Use wide spatula to flip patties.

Serve
Serve salmon cakes over bed of greens with lemon wedges.

Sweet Potato Chard Wraps

Preparation: 30 min.

Serves: 4

Ingredients

- 1 large shallot
- 2 cloves of garlic
- 1 lime
- 1 can black beans, or 2 cups cooked beans
- 1 large sweet potato
- 1 bunch chard
- 1 avocado
- 1/4 cup cilantro

- 1 Tbs coconut oil
- 2 tsp curry powder
- 1/2 tsp turmeric
- 2 tsp cumin
- 1/2 tsp chili powder (optional)
- Salt and pepper to taste
- 1/2 cup water

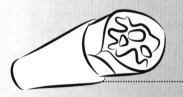

*F*or a healthy and satisfying take on tacos, I have added sweet potato and substituted chard for taco shells. Sweet potatoes are prized for their antioxidant and anti-inflammatory properties as well as their high levels of beta-carotene, which helps protect cells from damage. Dark green leafy vegetables such as chard contain high levels of B vitamins, which are vital for maintaining neurologic function. Rich in slow-digesting carbohydrates, protein, and fiber, beans are considered a low Glycemic Index food which helps regulate blood sugar levels.

Prep
Peel and finely chop shallot and garlic. Juice lime. Rinse and drain beans. Grate sweet potato, leaving skin on. Cut the chard leaves from the stems; set aside. Finely chop chard stems. Peel, pit, and slice avocado. Roughly chop cilantro.

Filling
Saute garlic and shallot in coconut oil until shallot is soft. Add spices, and saute a few minutes longer, stirring constantly.
   Add sweet potatoes, chard stems, lime juice, and water; cover and simmer until sweet potatoes are nearly done, adding more water if necessary and stirring occasionally. Add in black beans, and continue to cook until beans are warm and liquid is gone.

Wraps
Rinse chard leaves, but don't dry them.
   Heat a dry skillet, place leaves individually or a few at a time in skillet, and cover. They will steam with the water left on the leaves from rinsing. Watch them carefully; it only takes about a minute!

Serve
Wrap a few spoonfuls of the filling in each leaf. Garnish with avocado and cilantro.

Zesty Chicken Patties

Preparation: 15 min.

Serves: 4

Ingredients

A delightful retreat from the bland chicken patties of yesterday! Replete with antioxidants and anti-inflammatories, these zesty chicken patties are filled with healing properties that will satisfy even the most discerning of palates. They are bright, colorful, and pack a tasty punch. Make a big batch on the weekend for a week's worth of easy lunches. Rolling the patties in hemp seeds provides a visual and textural surprise, as well as an added dose of Omega-3 fatty acids.

- 2 garlic cloves
- 2/3 cup cilantro
- 3 green onions
- 1 tsp fresh ginger
- 1 pound ground chicken
- 1 tsp red chile powder (or to taste)
- 1 tsp fish sauce
- ½ tsp Himalayan salt
- ½ tsp pepper
- ½ lime
- ½ tsp turmeric
- 2 Tbs coconut oil
- 2 Tbs hemp seeds

Prep
Peel and finely chop the garlic. Finely chop the cilantro and onions. Grate the ginger. Mix garlic, cilantro, onions, and ginger along with the chicken, chile, fish sauce, salt, pepper, lime juice, and turmeric. Form into patties, rub lightly with oil, and roll edges in hemp seeds.

Saute or grill about eight minutes on each side, or until done.

- Mixed salad greens for serving

Serve
Serve over a bed of your favorite greens

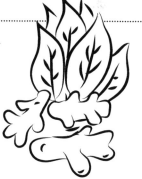

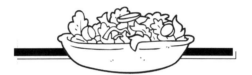

Salads

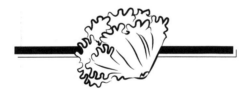

Avocado and Watercress Salad

Preparation: 15 min.

Serves: 4

*T*his lovely, bright salad is a great introduction to the peppery and lovely watercress, a humble, cruciferous, aquatic green leafy vegetable which has been eaten since ancient times. Long considered food for the lower classes, it has recently regained popularity because of its high nutritional value. Watercress provides numerous health benefits, including cancer prevention, lowering blood pressure, and healthy bone support. It is rich in vitamins, minerals, iron, and calcium. The folate it contains has been shown, among other benefits, to improve cognition and verbal fluency—good news for prevention of cognitive decline!

Ingredients

- 6 cups watercress
- 1 avocado
- 1/4 cup sweet onion
- 1 pomegranate
- 1/2 cup slivered almonds

Prep
Prepare the watercress by rinsing in cold water, then removing any yellowed or limp leaves and trimming excess stems. Peel and slice the avocado, finely slice the onion, and seed the pomegranate.

Toast the almonds in a dry skillet over medium heat, stirring frequently.

- 1/4 cup rice vinegar
- 4 tsp tamari
- 1 tsp honey
- 3 Tbs extra virgin olive oil

Dressing
Whisk together vinegar, tamari, and honey until blended, then stir in oil.

Salad
Toss watercress with enough dressing to coat, stir in onion, pomegranate seeds, and almonds.

Serve
Divide watercress among plates, garnish with avocado slices.

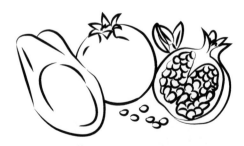

Beet and Yogurt Salad

Preparation: 20 min. active, 3–4 hours for baking and marinating

Serves: 4

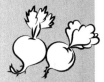

Ingredients

This is a beautiful, warm salad. Try a mix of golden and red beets for more vibrant color. Using both the roots and the greens, this salad makes full use of the beet. The greens are the most nutrient-rich part of the beet and are known as dark green leafy vegetables. They provide even more magnesium, and a better calcium-to-magnesium ratio than other members of the group. Beet greens are also high in vitamins K, A, and C as well as iron.

- 4 medium size beets
- Extra virgin olive oil
- 1/4 cup shallots
- 4 garlic cloves
- 2 Tbs mint
- 2 Tbs cilantro

Prep
Remove greens from beets and set aside. Drizzle whole beets with extra virgin olive oil and roast in a foil packet at 350 degrees until tender, 25 to 60 minutes, depending on the size of the beets. Peel and chop into bite-sized pieces or slices.

While beets are baking, prepare the rest of the ingredients. Peel and dice shallots. Peel and finely chop garlic. Chop mint, cilantro, and beet greens.

- 1½ Tbs sherry vinegar
- 1 tsp molasses
- 2 Tbs extra virgin olive oil

Marinade
Stir together the vinegar, molasses, olive oil, and salt and pepper to taste. Toss with the warm beets and marinate for 2 to 3 hours at room temperature or in the refrigerator.

- 1/4 tsp mustard seeds
- 1/4 tsp cumin seeds

Salad
Heat 2 tablespoons extra virgin olive oil over medium heat, add shallots and half the garlic. Saute until onion is translucent. Add mustard seeds, stirring frequently. When they begin to pop, add the cumin seeds. Add in beet greens, and saute for a few more minutes, stirring frequently.

- 1/2 cup plain goat yogurt
- 1/4 tsp Himalayan salt
- 1/4 tsp freshly ground pepper

Dressing
Mash the remainder of the garlic and salt. Stir into the yogurt. Add pepper. Drain the beets, saving some of the marinade to stir into the yogurt. Add beets to dressing and toss gently to coat.

- 2 Tbs pine nuts

Serve
Make a bed of beet greens on the plates. Place the beets in the center of the greens and top with pine nuts, mint and cilantro.

Carrot and Black-Eyed Pea Salad

Preparation: 45 min.

Serves: 4

Ingredients

K ale is one of the healthiest vegetables, and you can't go wrong with the other nutrient-rich ingredients in this salad. It is sweet and tangy, providing a wealth of taste sensations as well as an abundance of vitamins, minerals, fiber, and protein. Black-eyed peas are a good source of soluble fiber, potassium, folate, manganese, and beta-carotene.

- 1/2 cup cashews
- 1 cup dried black-eyed peas

Prep

Chop cashews and toast them in a dry skillet over medium-high heat, stirring frequently. Remove from heat and set aside.

If using dried black-eyed peas, cook according to package directions to make 2 cups cooked beans. Drain, rinse, and set aside to cool. Substitute drained and rinsed canned beans if you prefer.

- 1 large garlic clove
- 1/2 inch ginger
- 1/2 cup extra virgin olive oil
- Juice of 2 limes
- 1 tsp turmeric
- 1 Tbs maple syrup
- 1 tsp ground cumin
- 1/2 tsp Himalayan salt
- 1/8 tsp cayenne pepper

Dressing

Mince garlic and grate ginger. Whisk together, along with olive oil, lime juice, turmeric, maple syrup, cumin, salt, and cayenne pepper. Set aside.

- 1/2 cup dried dates
- 4–6 carrots
- 1 bunch kale
- 1/3 cup fresh cilantro
- 1 avocado
- 1/2 cup goat feta or parmesan cheese

Salad

Chop dates into small pieces, being mindful of the pits. Shred enough carrots to make 1½ cups. Chop kale, including stems. Chop cilantro. Peel and dice avocado.

In a medium bowl, combine the carrots, black-eyed peas, dried dates, cashews, kale, and cilantro. Mix in dressing, and toss gently until everything is evenly coated. Toss in avocado and cheese. Serve immediately, or cover and refrigerate until ready to serve.

Kale and Beet Salad

Preparation: 20 min.

Serves: 4

This dazzling salad is a big hit with guests and at potlucks. It's bright, colorful, and utterly appealing. For added flair, consider slicing the beets or cutting them into fine matchsticks. Beets are mighty yet humble root vegetables which contain powerful antioxidants and anti-inflammatories. Like other cruciferous vegetables, it has a high concentration of the antioxidants carotenoids and flavonoids, which have been shown to prevent cancer. Kale is also an excellent source of vitamin K, a critical nutrient in supporting the body's anti-inflammatory process. This is a wonderful salad for any point along your journey to better health.

Ingredients

- 1/2 cup pumpkin seeds
- 1 bunch kale
- 1 large golden beet
- 1 large red beet
- 1/2 red onion
- 2 Tbs fresh dill
- 1 clove garlic
- 1/2 lemon

Prep
Toast pumpkin seeds in a dry skillet over medium heat, stirring frequently. Separate kale leaves from stems; slice leaves and stems. Peel and dice beets. Chop red onion and dill. Mince or finely slice garlic. Juice lemon to make 1 Tbs juice.

- Himalayan salt
- Freshly ground black pepper
- 3 Tbs red wine vinegar

Marinade
Place kale, beets, and onion in a large mixing bowl, and season liberally with salt and pepper. Mix and top with the vinegar. Set aside. (This can be done up to a couple of hours in advance.)

Salad
Whisk together the oil, garlic, dill, and lemon juice. Toss the oil mixture with the kale, beets, and onion. Add feta and pumpkin seeds. Mix and serve.

- 6 Tbs extra virgin olive oil
- 1/2 cup crumbled feta

Serve
Serve the salad topped with feta and pumpkin seeds

Quinoa Salad with Black Beans

Preparation: 30 min.

Serves: 4

*T*his dish is visually appealing and very nourishing. In addition to antioxidants, each cup of black beans provides 15 grams of protein and fiber. Black beans also contain small amounts of Omega-3 fatty acids that still are about three times as much as in other beans. The cilantro not only adds depth to the flavor but also has been shown to aid digestion and soothe inflammation. The cumin enhances the taste of the salad while promoting the assimilation of other foods. You can substitute or add a variety of other ingredients such as dark green leafy vegetables and scallions.

Ingredients

- 1½ cups quinoa
- 1 can black beans
- 3 cups chicken broth
- 1 avocado
- 2 carrots
- 3 dates
- 1/2 cup cilantro
- 2½ limes

- 1½ Tbs apple cider vinegar
- 1 tsp cumin, or more to taste
- 1/3 cup extra virgin olive oil
- 1/4 tsp salt

- 1/3 cup goat cheese crumbles

Prep

Rinse and drain quinoa and beans. In a saucepan, bring broth to a boil, add quinoa, cover, and simmer on low heat until all the water is absorbed and quinoa is tender, about ten to fifteen minutes. Allow to cool.

Peel and chop avocado. Grate carrots. Chop dates and cilantro. Juice limes.

Dressing

In a small bowl, combine lime juice, vinegar, cumin, oil, and salt; whisk.

Salad

In a large bowl, mix cooked quinoa, beans, avocado, carrots, dates, and cilantro. Pour dressing over quinoa mixture, sprinkle in crumbled goat cheese, and toss gently.

Serve

Dish onto plates, enjoy!

Spicy Salmon Slaw

Preparation: 30 min.

Serves: 4

This peppy slaw is a perfect accompaniment to salmon's natural sweetness. Ginger and turmeric augment the salmon's many benefits and give it a bit of a kick. Salmon provides abundant Omega-3 fatty acids, which are vital to cell wall and nerve cell integrity—a great help to maintaining cognitive function. Ginger and turmeric are powerful anti-inflammatories, and turmeric provides the minerals manganese, iron, copper, and potassium, in addition to fiber and vitamin B6. Carrots are important antioxidants, as well as providing vitamins A, C, K, and B6.

Ingredients

- Sprouted rice
- 1 pound red cabbage
- 1 pound carrots
- 1/2 cup fresh cilantro
- 3 limes

Prep
Cook rice according to package directions, enough for four servings. Shred cabbage. Coarsely grate carrot. Chop cilantro. Juice 2 limes. Cut another lime into wedges.

- 2 Tbs olive oil
- Lime juice
- 1/2 tsp Himalayan salt
- 1/2 tsp ground pepper

Dressing
Whisk oil, lime juice, salt, and pepper in a small bowl.

Slaw
In a large bowl, toss cabbage, carrots, and cilantro with dressing. Mix well, and refrigerate until ready to serve.

- 1 tsp turmeric
- 1 tsp ginger
- 4 salmon filets

Salmon
Stir turmeric and ginger together. Gently rub salmon with spice mixture. Grill six to eight minutes per side, or until salmon reaches desired temperature.

Serve
Divide slaw among plates; serve with sliced salmon and rice.

Sweet Potato Salad

Preparation: 20 min., plus 2 hours to set.

Serves: 4

*M*y take on the traditional potato salad pairs the natural sweetness of cinnamon with the tanginess of Dijon mustard. Letting the salad set up in the refrigerator for as long as twenty-four hours before serving allows the flavors to mingle perfectly. Cinnamon is one of humanity's oldest known spices, dating back to at least 2700 B.C. Prized for its medicinal properties in ancient China, it is now used the world over. Cinnamon is an excellent source of manganese, which helps grow strong bones, maintains skin integrity, helps to control blood sugar, and protects against free radical damage.

Ingredients

- 1/2 cup frozen edamame
- 3 pounds sweet potatoes
- 1/2 inch ginger
- 1/2 lime
- 1/2 small red onion
- 3 stalks celery
- 1/4 cup fresh dill

Prep
Thaw and shell edamame. Dice sweet potatoes. Grate ginger. Juice lime. Thinly slice onion and celery. Finely chop dill.

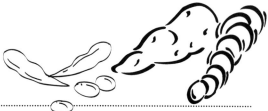

Stovetop
In a medium saucepan with a steamer basket and 1 inch of water, steam sweet potatoes until tender, ten to fifteen minutes. Allow to cool.

- 2 tablespoons Dijon mustard
- 1/8 tsp cinnamon
- 1/4 tsp Himalayan salt
- 1/4 tsp black pepper

Dressing
Whisk together lime juice, mustard, ginger, cinnamon, salt, and pepper.

Salad
Combine onion, edamame, celery, and dill in a large bowl. Stir in sweet potatoes, and toss with dressing. Cover and refrigerate at least two, and up to twenty-four, hours.

Thai Beef Salad

Preparation: 20 min.

Serves: 4

Ingredients

- 2 Thai chile peppers
- 2 cloves garlic
- 2 inches fresh ginger
- 1/2 cup cilantro
- 1/2 cup basil
- 1/2 cup red onion
- 1 cucumber
- 2 tomatoes
- 1 pound flank steak
- 4 limes
- 1 head romaine lettuce

- 1/4 cup tamari
- 1/4 cup fish sauce
- 2 Tbs blackstrap molasses

- 1/2 tsp toasted sesame oil

- 1 Tbs sesame oil

*M*olasses adds a note of complexity to this bright, beautiful salad. Feel free to adjust the amount of chile peppers for individual tastes. These peppers, which owe their heat to capsaicin, are in the nightshade family, like tomatoes. While I don't often recommend nightshades, in moderation, they offer plenty of health benefits. If your body does not react well to them, by all means, leave them out.

Prep
Seed and chop chile peppers. Peel and roughly chop garlic and ginger. Chop cilantro. Cut basil into ribbons. Thinly slice onion crosswise. Slice cucumber and tomatoes. Cut steak slices across the grain. Juice limes. Tear romaine leaves into bite-sized pieces.

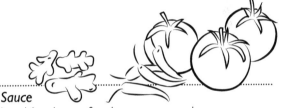

Sauce
In a blender or food processor, pulse peppers, garlic, and ginger until finely chopped. Add tamari, fish sauce, molasses, cilantro, and lime juice; process until well combined. Separate 1/3 cup of mixture for salad dressing; set aside.

Dressing
Whisk reserved sauce with sesame oil to make salad dressing.

Salad
In a large bowl, toss romaine, basil, onion, cucumber, and tomatoes with salad dressing.

Steak
Heat oil in a large skillet over medium heat. Saute steak over medium-high heat for 1 minute per side, and toss with remaining sauce.

Serve
Divide salad among dishes; top with steak slices.

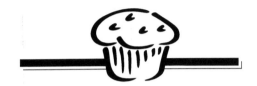

Sweets and Snacks

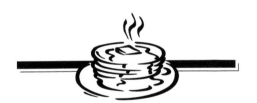

Amaranth Pancakes

Preparation: 15 min.

Serves: 2

*T*hese pancakes are nutty and substantial. Even though they're gluten-free, they have a delicious, cake-like texture that will carry you until lunch. Cultivated by the Aztecs 8,000 years ago, amaranth was a major staple of ancient diets in Mexico and Central America. It is now used throughout the world and provides many health benefits. It is the only grain with a documented vitamin C content, and is high in protein, calcium, iron, phosphorus, carotenoids, and fiber, as well as antioxidant and anti-inflammatory properties.

Ingredients

Prep
Grate ginger root. Melt coconut oil. Juice lemon.

- 1/4 inch ginger root
- 2 tsp coconut oil
- 1 lemon

Dry Ingredients
Mix dry ingredients in a large bowl, using a wire whisk, until well combined. Reserve.

- 1 cup amaranth flour
- 1/2 cup arrowroot powder
- 1/2 cup almond meal
- 1 tsp baking soda
- 1 tsp ground cinnamon
- 1/4 tsp cloves
- 1/4 tsp salt

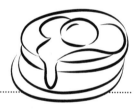

Liquids
In a separate bowl, using a wire whisk, beat egg until it is lemony in color. Stir in ginger root, lemon juice, coconut oil, and molasses; mix well.

- 1 egg
- 2 Tbs blackstrap molasses
- water as needed for consistency

Process
Make a well in the middle of the dry ingredients. Gently pour liquid into the well. Using a wooden spoon, go around the outside edge of the dry ingredients to gently pull the dry into the liquid. Mix like this as gently as you can, just until all the ingredients are wet but some bits of dry remain.

Drop the batter onto a lightly oiled griddle or frying pan, heated to medium-high. When edges begin to bubble, flip and cook other side.

Chocolate Date Balls

Preparation: 10 min., plus 1 hour to freeze.

Serves: Makes 2 dozen balls.

Ingredients

- 2 Tbs pine nuts
- 1 cup shredded coconut
- 2 cups dates
- 2 cups almond meal
- 1/2 cup almond butter
- 1 Tbs chia seeds
- 1 tsp cinnamon
- 1 cup unsweetened cocoa powder
- 1/4 cup maple syrup
- 1/4 cup water
- Additional ground nuts or coconut flakes for rolling, optional

These cookies are a great snack to carry with you on busy days. Make a big batch and keep them in the freezer for a quick chocolate fix that is packed with vitamins and minerals. Dates have been a favorite food since ancient times, and are grown in arid regions throughout the world. They are easily digested, and have antioxidant and anti-inflammatory properties, being high in fiber, vitamins, and minerals—particularly iron, B vitamins, and vitamins A and K.

Prep

If you wish to, toast the pine nuts or coconut in a dry skillet over medium-high heat, stirring constantly until toasted.

Chop dates (being careful of the pits), and dust with almond meal. Mix with the other ingredients in a large bowl. You will probably want to use your hands or a food processor to mix well, as the batter can be hard to stir. Use additional water or almond meal to improve the texture if necessary. Form into 1-inch balls, and roll in the ground nuts or coconut flakes if desired.

Freeze at least one hour before serving.

Energy Bars

Preparation: 20 min., plus 12 hours inactive.

Serves: 8

Ingredients

*T*hese energy bars are a perfect take-along treat for those busy days! They have a lovely amount of sweetness without being sticky or messy. Chia seeds are high in Omega-3 fatty acids. Dates have a lot of fiber and vitamins A and K as well as minerals such as calcium, iron, and phosphorus. Sunflower seeds are an excellent source of vitamin E, the body's primary fat-soluble antioxidant. Vitamin E has significant anti-inflammatory effects.

- 1/2 cup dried dates

Prep
Chop dates; be careful of the pits!

- 2 cups raw almonds
- 1/2 cup maple syrup
- 2/3 cup coconut oil
- 2 tsp vanilla
- 1 tsp Himalayan salt
- 1/2 cup sunflower seeds
- 1 tsp cinnamon
- 1/2 tsp nutmeg
- 4 cups oats
- 1 cup shredded coconut
- 3/4 cup sliced almonds
- 1/4 cup chia seeds
- 1/3 cup dark chocolate chips

Bars
Line a 9" × 9" baking pan with wax paper.

In a blender or food processor, combine 2 cups raw almonds, maple syrup, coconut oil, vanilla, and salt. In a separate bowl, combine remaining ingredients. Stir in almond mixture. Spread into pan and press evenly. Let sit at room temperature 8–12 hours or overnight. Cut into bars.

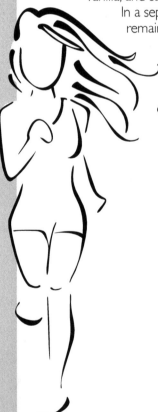

Granola

Preparation: 1½ hours

Serves: 12

Ingredients

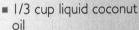

- 1½ cups walnuts, pecans, or almonds
- 1/2 cup dried dates (optional)
- 2 Tbs almond flour

- 1/3 cup liquid coconut oil
- 1/4 cup maple syrup
- 1 tsp vanilla extract
- 3½ cups rolled oats
- 1/2 cup pumpkin seeds
- 1 Tbs hemp seeds
- 1 tsp pine nuts
- 1/3 cup chunky salted almond butter
- 1 tsp cinnamon
- 1/2 tsp ground nutmeg
- 1/4 tsp ground cardamom
- 1 Tbs chia seeds
- 1/2 cup shredded unsweetened coconut

*H*omemade granola is a delicious, economical, and healthy alternative to store-bought snacks. Take a couple of handfuls along on a hike or as a nourishing between-meal snack. Surprisingly easy to make, granola is versatile and can be made ahead and stored in the freezer. Oats have many health benefits, including lowering cholesterol and the risk of cardiovascular disease. They also enhance the immune response to infection, stabilize blood sugar, and lower the risk of Type 2 diabetes. Chia and hemp seeds are an abundant plant source of Omega-3.

Prep
Chop nuts and dates. Toss dates with almond flour.

Granola
In a small bowl, mix liquid ingredients. In a large bowl, mix dry ingredients; stir well. Pour wet ingredients into dry, stirring frequently.

Spray rimmed baking sheet with coconut oil, spread granola evenly on sheet. Bake at 275 degrees for one hour, stirring every fifteen minutes. When mixture is cool, transfer to bowl and add chia seeds and shredded coconut.

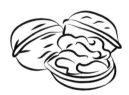

Serve
Enjoy granola by itself or with plain goat yogurt or your favorite milk. Excess can be frozen.

Nourishing Smoothie

Preparation: 10 min.

Serves: 2

Ingredients

*T*his smoothie makes a nourishing and energizing snack rich in vitamins, antioxidants, and fiber. Blueberries, one of the richest sources of antioxidants around, are also a good source of fiber, which has been shown to improve digestive health and prevent constipation. Blueberries also have useful amounts of vitamin C, potassium, calcium, and magnesium, and raspberries contain calcium, fiber, and folate. Berries contain powerful antioxidant phytochemicals that decrease inflammation.

- 2 ripe bananas
- 1/2 can (7 oz.) coconut milk or milk of your choice
- 1 cup plain kefir (easily digestible) or plain yogurt
- 2 Tbs almond butter
- 1 Tbs ground flaxseed
- 1 cup fresh or frozen berries (blueberries and/or raspberries recommended)
- 2 cups ice

Prep
Combine all ingredients in blender, and blend until smooth. For a little extra flavor, add a few drops of vanilla extract. If desired, add honey to sweeten.

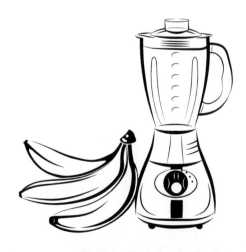

Pumpkin Walnut Pancakes

Preparation: 45 min.

Serves: 4

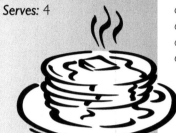

*P*ancakes are always a big hit with guests and children. Additionally, they store well and can be made ahead for an easy weekday breakfast. But don't underestimate the potential of pancakes for dinner! Alongside your favorite steamed veggies, or a light soup, these pancakes make a satisfying dinner. They are packed with Omega-3 fatty acids.

For a twist, try using another winter squash in place of the pumpkin. Simply cut the squash in half, seed, and spread coconut oil or butter on the cut half, then bake, cut side down on a baking dish at 350 degrees for 45 minutes. Spoon out the flesh and mash or blend and use in place of the pumpkin puree.

Ingredients

- 1/2 cup walnuts

- 1/2 cup almond flour
- 2 Tbs coconut flour
- 1 Tbs chia seeds
- 1/8 tsp salt
- 2 tsp cinnamon
- 1/2 tsp ginger, ground
- 1/2 tsp nutmeg, ground
- 1/4 tsp baking soda
- 1/2 cup pumpkin puree
- 3 eggs
- 2 Tbs maple syrup
- 1/2 tsp vanilla extract
- Coconut oil for cooking pancakes

Prep
Chop walnuts. Heat a pancake griddle to medium, or 350 degrees.

Pancakes
Combine dry ingredients in a bowl. Whisk together wet ingredients in a small bowl. Add wet to dry ingredients, stirring just long enough to mix. Some lumps will remain in the batter.

Add enough coconut oil to the pan to grease the center.

Pour batter in approximately 1/4 cupsful onto pan and spread out into pancake shape. (The batter will be a bit thick and need some help to form a circle.)

Cook for about 3–4 minutes on the first side, carefully flip and cook for another 1–2 minutes on the second side. Repeat with remaining batter, adding more coconut oil to the pan as needed.

Serve
Serve along with slices of your favorite fruit and pure maple syrup or applesauce.

Quinoa Pumpkin Muffins

Preparation: 10 min. to prepare, 40 min. to cook

Serves: 6

These muffins are delicious and nutritious, and make a nourishing, energy-sustaining snack food. The soluble fiber of the dates helps regulate blood sugar levels while providing a rich source of B vitamins, potassium, and magnesium. The walnuts are an excellent source of antioxidants and help reduce inflammation; they are one of the highest vegetarian food sources of Omega-3 fatty acids. Additionally, the cinnamon not only boosts the flavor of the muffins but also has been shown to help lower blood sugar, and a half-teaspoon a day of this common spice has been found to lower LDL cholesterol. For those who are gluten-free, try experimenting with gluten-free flours such as coconut flour. While I don't often recommend spelt flour, once in a while, it's okay.

Ingredients

- Quinoa
- 1/3 cup chopped dates
- 1/3 cup walnuts

Prep
Cook quinoa according to package directions, enough to make 1/2 cup cooked grain. Chop dates and walnuts.

Preheat oven to 350 degrees. Prep muffin tins with liners or oil.

- 1 cup spelt flour or flour of your choice
- 1 egg
- 2 Tbs chia seeds
- 1/2 tsp cinnamon
- 1/4 tsp nutmeg
- 1/4 tsp cloves (optional)
- 1/2 tsp salt
- 1/2 tsp vanilla extract
- 1½ cups pumpkin puree
- 3 Tbs coconut oil
- 2 tsp baking powder
- 1–2 Tbs maple syrup (optional)

Muffins
Combine all the ingredients in a mixing bowl; blend well. Pour batter evenly into muffin tins. Bake thirty to forty minutes, or until the muffins are cooked through.

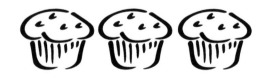

Serve
Allow to cool before enjoying.

Superfood Pudding

Preparation: 15 minutes plus 12 hours to set up

Serves: 6

*T*his lightly sweet pudding, reminiscent of tapioca, makes a delicious breakfast or snack. It is easy to prepare, though it does need to rest for several hours or overnight. Chia and blueberries are both considered "superfoods" because of their health benefits. Blueberries are high in vitamins and have anti-inflammatory properties. And there is promising new evidence that they can improve memory and slow down or postpone the onset of cognitive problems. Blueberries also are rich in antioxidant nutrients, which help maintain smoothly functioning nerve cells and healthy cognitive function. Chia has an abundance of Omega-3 fats as well as being high in calcium and manganese.

Ingredients

- 1/2 cup sliced almonds

Prep
Toast almonds in a dry skillet over medium heat, stirring frequently; remove from heat and allow to cool.

- 1 can coconut milk
- 2 cups plain Greek yogurt
- 3 Tbs plus 6 tsp maple syrup
- 1/2 cup chia seeds
- 2 tsp vanilla
- 1/2 tsp Himalayan salt
- 2 pints blueberries

Pudding
Mix the coconut milk, Greek yogurt, 3 tablespoons maple syrup, chia, vanilla, and Himalayan salt. Cover and refrigerate for eight to twelve hours, stirring occasionally.

Mix the blueberries with the remaining 6 teaspoons maple syrup. Stir in almonds.

Serve
Serve in dishes with alternating layers of chia mixture and berries.

Stir-Frys, Hashes, and Curries

Beef Stir-Fry

Preparation: 30 min.

Serves: 4

*H*ave you ever eaten cooked radishes? They are a surprising addition to this stir-fry, which also uses the often-overlooked radish greens. As members of the cruciferous vegetable family, radishes protect against cancer by providing phytonutrients, fiber, vitamins, and minerals. The sweetness of the onion is a nice balance to the peppery radishes. Stir-frys are great because they are unendingly versatile and cook up rather quickly. Chopping extra veggies that you keep in the fridge can save time for another meal, since they'll be ready to stir-fry any time!

Ingredients

- 2 cups sprouted rice or quinoa
- 1 bunch radishes
- 1/2 inch fresh ginger
- 2 cloves garlic
- 1/2 cup yellow onion
- 1/2 pound sirloin
- 1/2 tsp curry powder
- 1/8 tsp Himalayan salt
- 1/8 tsp black pepper
- 1/2 tsp turmeric

- 2 Tbs butter
- 1 Tbs honey
- 2 Tbs tamari
- 1 Tbs balsamic vinegar
- 1 cup snow peas
- 1/4 tsp salt

Prep

Cook rice or quinoa according to package directions.

Cut radishes into quarters, or eighths if they are large. Save greens, rinse well, and set aside. Peel and thinly slice ginger and garlic. Finely chop onion. Thinly slice sirloin.

In a medium bowl, mix curry powder, salt, pepper, and turmeric. Toss with sirloin, mix well to coat evenly.

Stir-Fry

Heat 1 tablespoon butter in a large skillet over medium-high heat. Add sirloin in an even layer, and cook undisturbed until browned on bottom, about one minute. Flip and cook for an additional thirty seconds. Remove from skillet and set aside.

Add another tablespoon of butter to the skillet, reduce heat to low, and cook ginger, garlic, onion, and radishes, stirring frequently, until onion is soft, about six minutes. Add 1 tablespoon honey, and increase heat to medium; cook until radishes are glazed, about two minutes. Add tamari and balsamic vinegar, and simmer until thickened, about two minutes. Add radish greens, snow peas and 1/4 teaspoon salt. Continue to cook, stirring frequently, until greens are wilted. Toss in beef to rewarm.

Serve

Serve over a bed of sprouted rice or quinoa.

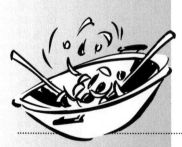

Butternut Squash Curry

Preparation: 30 min.

Serves: 4

This gentle curry is a combination of sweet and mild heat. In addition to balancing the squash's natural sweetness, the curry paste provides antioxidants and cancer-fighting benefits. If you prefer a more-robust curry taste, feel free to substitute with a stronger curry paste. Winter squash, such as butternut, provides many minerals and other nutrients such as B vitamins, potassium, and magnesium, as well as Omega-3 and fiber.

Ingredients

- 1 cup finely chopped shallot
- 2 cloves thinly sliced garlic
- 2-pound butternut squash
- 1 can chickpeas
- 1/2 cup cilantro
- 2 cups quinoa

Prep
Peel and slice shallot and garlic. Peel and remove seeds from one large butternut squash; chop into bite-sized chunks. Rinse and drain one can chickpeas. Chop cilantro.

Cook quinoa according to package instructions.

- 1 Tbs coconut oil
- 1 can coconut milk
- 3 Tbs mild curry paste, or more to taste
- 1 tsp salt

Curry
In a large pot over medium heat, melt coconut oil. Add shallot and garlic, and cook, stirring frequently, until shallot is soft, about three minutes. Add coconut milk, curry paste, and salt; bring to a boil. Add squash; return to boil.

Reduce heat and simmer, uncovered, fifteen minutes or until squash is tender. Stir in chickpeas and cilantro; continue to cook until warmed through.

- 1 lime

Serve
Slice lime into wedges; serve curry with a squeeze of lime over a bed of quinoa. .

Cauliflower Hash

Preparation: 30 min.

Serves: 4

Ingredients

- 1 cauliflower
- 1 bunch green onions
- 1 small zucchini
- 3 cloves garlic
- 1 inch ginger
- 1/4 cup cilantro
- 1 lime

- 2 Tbs coconut oil
- 1 pound ground turkey
- 1 tsp turmeric
- 1 tsp ground cumin
- 1/4 tsp black pepper
- 1/2 tsp Himalayan salt

*T*his beautiful and balanced dish shines for its versatility. Serve it for a weekend brunch or a weeknight dinner; it is guaranteed to delight your family and guests alike! Cauliflower makes an intriguing substitute for potatoes, offering abundant fiber, vitamins, and minerals without the carbs. It has abundant amounts of vitamins C and K and beta-carotene. Cauliflower is a member of the cruciferous family of vegetables, which is known for its cancer-fighting properties. Research has indicated that combining cauliflower with curcumin (the active ingredient in turmeric) may help prevent prostate cancer. Cauliflower is anti-inflammatory and antioxidant rich. Robust flavors and textures make this an exciting as well as a healing dish.

Prep
Core and grate the cauliflower, dice the onions and zucchini, peel and mince or chop the garlic, and grate the ginger. Chop the cilantro, and slice the lime into wedges.

Hash
Heat 1 tablespoon coconut oil in a large skillet over medium heat. Add cauliflower, garlic, and onion. Cook, stirring occasionally, for eight to ten minutes. Remove from pan and set aside.

Heat remaining oil, and cook turkey along with the turmeric, cumin, pepper, salt, and ginger for five minutes. Add zucchini and cook a further three to five minutes.

Serve
Toss turkey mixture with cauliflower and cilantro, and serve with a squeeze of lime.

Festival Chicken Stir-Fry

Preparation: 45 min.

Serves: 4

*T*he secret to a good stir-fry is to be prepared with all the ingredients chopped, measured, and at the ready when you begin heating the oil. This recipe uses pre-cooked chicken, so you don't have to worry about timing the cooking of the raw meat. I like stir-frys because they are an easy way to incorporate beneficial spices that taste good. Plus, kids like it, and it makes for great leftovers. Coconut aminos are a product made from the sap of the coconut tree. They are a sustainable, soy-free alternative to soy sauce for those who prefer to avoid soy. This recipe is packed full of turmeric, a potent anti-inflammatory which has been used in Chinese and Indian medicine for centuries. Growing evidence demonstrates that turmeric offers protection against neurodegenerative diseases.

Ingredients

- Sprouted rice or quinoa
- 1 shallot
- 2 cups shiitake mushrooms
- 2 cups broccoli florets
- 3 large carrots
- 6 cloves garlic
- 1½-inch piece ginger
- 2 cups chicken, cooked
- 1 lime

- 2 Tbs coconut oil
- 1/2 cup coconut aminos
- 1/2 tsp Himalayan salt
- 1 Tbs turmeric
- 1/2 cup sugar snap peas

Prep

Cook quinoa or rice according to package directions to make 2 cups of cooked grains.

Finely chop shallots. Roughly chop mushrooms and broccoli. Thinly slice carrots. Mince or finely chop garlic; grate ginger. Shred or roughly chop chicken meat. Slice lime into wedges.

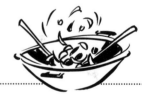

Stir-Fry

Heat coconut oil in a wok or large skillet. Add shallots, and cook one minute, stirring frequently. Add mushrooms; cook two minutes, stirring frequently. Add garlic and ginger, then carrots and broccoli; cook three minutes, stirring frequently. Stir in coconut aminos, salt, and turmeric. Add peas and chicken; cook long enough to warm chicken.

Serve

Serve over rice or quinoa with lime wedges.

Curried Quinoa and Veggies

Preparation: 45 min.

Serves: 4

Ingredients

- 1 cup quinoa
- 1-inch piece ginger

- 1 Tbs coconut oil
- 1 chopped shallot
- 2 diced carrots
- 1 Tbs green curry
  paste
- 1 tsp turmeric
- 2½ cups chicken stock
- 1 can coconut milk
- 1/2 tsp salt
- 1/4 tsp pepper

- 1 handful fresh peas

*T*his one-dish, delicious curry is versatile and a hit with the children. Serve as a side dish, or make it a meal by stirring in cooked chicken pieces at the end. It also makes a fine breakfast; simply add an egg or other protein source on top, and enjoy! Curry dishes are a great way to incorporate the healing spices turmeric and ginger, which foster brain health.

Prep
Rinse quinoa, soak for fifteen minutes in cold water, and drain. Grate the ginger.

Curry
Heat coconut oil in a large saucepan over medium heat. Saute until the shallot is translucent. Add ginger and carrots; saute a few minutes more. Add curry paste, turmeric, and a splash of stock. Increase heat, bring to a boil, then reduce heat and simmer for five minutes.

Add quinoa, coconut milk, and chicken stock. Increase heat, bring to a boil, then reduce heat, cover, and simmer for a further twenty minutes, or until quinoa is done.

Serve
Season with salt and pepper as desired, garnish with peas, and serve warm or at room temperature.

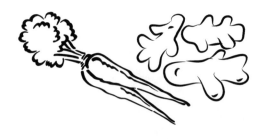

Curried Vegetable Saute

Preparation: 45 min.

Serves: 4

This is a mellow yet pleasing curry, a lovely way to introduce cabbage into the diet. This vegetable has numerous health benefits, not the least of which is the abundance of vitamins K and C. You'll notice that there are very few wheat-based products in this cookbook. Occasionally, though, I do like to offer couscous and other pastas for a bit of variety. Of course, if you are avoiding wheat or gluten, feel free to substitute quinoa. When paired with the bountiful benefits of the vegetables and healing spices in this recipe, couscous offers a delightful texture as well as the trace mineral selenium, which is essential for the body and difficult to find in food sources.

Ingredients

- Couscous
- 2 Tbs cashews
- 1 yellow onion
- 2 cups savoy cabbage
- 1/4 cup cilantro
- 1 sweet potato
- 4 dates
- 1 Tbs fresh ginger
- 3 cloves garlic
- 1 lime
- 1 can chickpeas

- 1 Tbs coconut oil
- 1 ½ tsp cumin
- 1 Tbs coriander
- 1 tsp turmeric
- 1/4 tsp black pepper
- 2 cups chicken or vegetable broth
- 1 can coconut milk

Prep
Cook couscous according to package directions to make four servings. Chop cashews, and toast them in a dry skillet over medium heat, stirring frequently. Set aside.

Chop onion, cabbage, and cilantro. Finely dice the sweet potato. Pit and chop dates. Grate ginger. Mince or press garlic. Cut lime into wedges. Rinse and drain chickpeas.

Curry
Saute onion, cumin, coriander, turmeric, and pepper in a large skillet over medium heat until onion begins to soften. Stir in cabbage, sweet potato, chickpeas, dates, ginger, and garlic. Saute an additional five minutes.

Add broth, reduce heat, and cover. Simmer until sweet potatoes are tender, about ten minutes, stirring occasionally. Stir in coconut milk, warm a few minutes longer.

Serve
Serve over couscous topped with cashews, cilantro, and a squeeze of lime.

Harvest Kuri Curry

*T*his tasty curry features red kuri, a beautiful winter squash. If red kuri is not available, feel free to substitute a winter squash of your choice. Red kuri is a naturally sweet, versatile squash that is great for baking and stuffing, as well as for use in stir-frys and curries. Kuri, like all winter squash, is high in vitamins A, B1, B2, and C, as well as the minerals calcium, potassium, and iron, and also is an excellent source of fiber. Winter squash have anti-inflammatory, antioxidant, and blood sugar benefits. Enjoy this beautiful dish on a crisp autumn day.

Preparation: 30 min. active, 45 min. to bake

Serves: 4

Ingredients

- 1/2 cup shredded coconut
- 1 medium red kuri squash
- 1 Tbs coconut oil
- 1 sweet onion
- 2 cloves garlic
- 2 inches fresh ginger
- 3 cups cauliflower
- 2 cups kale
- 1 lime
- Quinoa

- 2 Tbs coconut oil
- 2 tsp ground coriander
- 1/2 tsp salt
- 1 tsp turmeric
- 1 tsp ground mustard
- 1 tsp chile powder
- 1/2 tsp cayenne, or to taste
- 1/2 tsp cumin
- 1/4 tsp cardamon
- 2 cups chicken broth
- 1 can coconut milk

Prep

Preheat oven to 350 degrees. Toast coconut in a dry skillet over medium heat for two to three minutes, stirring constantly.

Cut squash in half; spread 1 tablespoon coconut oil on cut sides. Place in a baking dish cut sides down, and bake for thirty to forty-five minutes, or until tender.

While squash is baking, prep other ingredients. Peel and dice onion. Peel and press or mince garlic. Grate ginger. Chop cauliflower and kale. Juice lime.

Following package instructions, make enough quinoa for four servings.

Curry

Saute onion, garlic, and ginger in 2 tablespoons coconut oil in a dutch oven or soup pot over medium heat. When onion is translucent, add cauliflower, spices, and chicken broth. Simmer twenty minutes, or until cauliflower is al dente.

When squash is cooked, scoop out flesh and add to cauliflower. Stir in kale, coconut milk, and lime juice. Simmer until kale is bright green and tender, stirring occasionally.

Serve

Ladle over quinoa, and sprinkle toasted coconut on top.

Seafood Curry

Preparation: 20 min.

Serves: 4

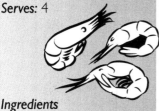

Ingredients

This beautiful curry cooks up quickly and will delight the whole family. Feel free to substitute salmon if allergies are an issue. Shrimp and scallops are readily available frozen year-round, and fresh seasonally. Shrimp contains anti-inflammatories and antioxidants, and is high in many vitamins and minerals, such as selenium, phosphorus, choline, iodine and vitamins B3, B6, B12, and E. It is also high in copper, a powerful antioxidant, and helps to maintain bone and tissue integrity.

Prep
Peel and thinly slice shallots. Peel and mince garlic and ginger. Juice lime. Dice carrots. Chop cilantro. Peel and de-vein shrimp. Cook quinoa according to package directions, enough for four servings.

- 2 large shallots
- 1 clove garlic
- 1 Tbs ginger
- 1/2 lime
- 2 medium carrots
- 1 cup cilantro
- 1 pound shrimp
- Quinoa

- 2 Tbs coconut oil
- 1/2 pound scallops
- 2 Tbs curry powder
- 1 tsp turmeric
- 2 stems lemon grass
- 1 Tbs maple syrup (optional)
- 1 can coconut milk
- 1/2 tsp Himalayan salt
- 1/4 tsp pepper
- 1/4 cup basil leaves
- 1/2 pound snow peas

Curry
In a saucepan over medium heat, saute shallots in coconut oil until soft. Add garlic, shrimp, scallops, curry powder, turmeric, and ginger, and cook for another few minutes, stirring frequently. Add lemon grass and carrots, and cook for a few minutes more, turning shrimp and scallops. Add maple syrup, coconut milk, salt, pepper, and lime juice, and bring to a simmer, cooking a further ten minutes. Stir in snow peas and basil.

Serve
Spoon curry over quinoa; garnish with cilantro.

Sweet Potato and Brussels Sprout

Preparation: 30 min.

Serves: 6

A favorite for Sunday brunch, this dish reheats well and is a good choice for a do-ahead weekday breakfast. Rosemary, reminiscent of evergreen trees, is prized for its anti-inflammatory properties and ability to aid digestion. Hash is also a good way to introduce brussels sprouts to eaters who may be unfamiliar with the myriad benefits of this lovely cruciferous vegetable. Like other members of the Brassica family, brussels sprouts have anti-inflammatory and antioxidant properties, and are also high in Omega-3 fatty acids.

Ingredients

- 3 eggs
- 2 sprigs rosemary
- 1 bunch green onions
- 1/2 pound brussels sprouts
- 2 portabella mushrooms
- 2 cloves garlic
- 2 inches fresh ginger
- 1 sweet potato
- 1 lemon

- 5 Tbs butter
- 1 Tbs turmeric

Prep

Separate eggs; set aside. Stem rosemary, and chop. Chop green onions, brussels sprouts, and mushrooms. Mince or press garlic. Press ginger. Peel and dice sweet potato. Juice lemon.

Sauce

Melt butter in a small saucepan over medium heat. Add rosemary and turmeric; cook for a minute or two. Remove from heat, and set aside.

To prepare the sauce, combine egg yolks with 1/4 cup of water and lemon juice in the top part of a double boiler or a small bowl that will fit over the saucepan of simmering water. Whisk mixture for several minutes, until it begins to thicken. Slowly add butter mixture, and continue to whisk until well mixed and sauce is thickened. Remove from heat and set aside.

Hash

Ingedients continued
- 4 eggs
- 2 Tbs coconut oil
- 2 tsp pepper
- 1/2 tsp salt

Hash
Saute onions, garlic, and ginger in a skillet over medium heat. While onions are cooking, heat 2 inches of water in a small saucepan or double boiler until simmering.

When onions are soft, add sweet potatoes and 1/4 cup water. Cover and cook a further eight to ten minutes, stirring frequently. When sweet potatoes are soft, add brussels sprouts and portabellas and cook four to five minutes longer, stirring frequently. Season with salt and pepper.

Prepare eggs as desired; if scrambling, mix in separated whites to avoid waste.

Serve
Divide hash among plates; serve each with an egg and sauce.

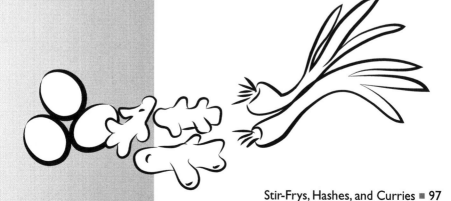

Baked Dishes

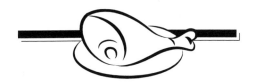

Ginger Turkey Cutlets

Preparation: 45 min.

Serves: 4

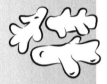

Ingredients

*T*his is an ambitious meal, definitely for a day when you have some time to spend in the kitchen. But your efforts will be well rewarded. Moist and flavorful, the turkey basks in a delicious and well-balanced sauce, and the meal contains many healing ingredients. Fennel, which is closely related to parsley, carrots, and dill, has played an important role in the traditional food culture of France and Italy dating back to ancient times. It supports many of the body's systems, and is particularly helpful for cardiovascular and colon health.

- 1 bunch green onions
- 2 bulbs fennel
- 1/4 pound shiitake mushrooms
- 1 bunch chard
- 2 cloves garlic
- 2 inches fresh ginger

Prep

Roughly chop onions, fennel, mushrooms, and chard. Peel and mince or press garlic. Grate ginger.

- 2 inches fresh ginger
- 2 limes
- 2 tsp toasted sesame oil
- 2 Tbs tamari
- 2 Tbs freshly ground black pepper
- 2 pounds turkey cutlets

Marinade

Grate ginger. Juice limes. In a small bowl, whisk together sesame oil, ginger, tamari, lime juice, and pepper. Marinate turkey in this mixture for one hour.

- 2¼ cups chicken broth
- 1 can coconut milk
- 2 cups uncooked sprouted rice
- 1/2 tsp salt

Rice

Meanwhile, start rice; bring 2¼ cups chicken broth and one can coconut milk to a boil over medium-high heat. Stir in rice and ½ teaspoon salt; cover, and reduce heat to low. Simmer twenty minutes or until rice is tender. Remove from heat; set aside.

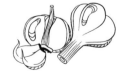

Ingredients continued
- 4 Tbs coconut flour
- 2 Tbs coconut oil

Turkey
When the marinating hour is nearly up, preheat oven to 350 degrees. Oil a large, ovenproof skillet, and heat over medium-high heat.

Remove turkey from marinade, discard marinade. Dust with coconut flour, and fry about one minute on each side.

Cover and bake until turkey reaches an internal temperature of 170 degrees, or about ten to fifteen minutes. Remove from pan, and set aside.

- 3 Tbs tamari
- 3 Tbs rice vinegar
- 1½ Tbs red wine vinegar
- 3 Tbs maple syrup
- 3 Tbs almond butter

Sauce
For the sauce, whisk together fresh ginger, tamari, rice vinegar, red wine vinegar, maple syrup, almond butter, and 2 tablespoons water. Set aside.

2 Tbs coconut oil
¼ cup chicken broth

Vegetables
Saute green onions and garlic in coconut oil over medium heat. Add fennel and mushrooms; continue to cook, stirring frequently until mushrooms soften. Add broth and chard, and cook until bright green. Toss veggies with some of the sauce.

Serve
Serve veggies and turkey over rice, with a drizzle of sauce.

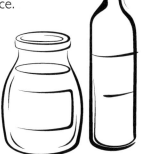

Golden Baked Chicken

Preparation: 20 min. active, 2 hours to marinate, and 45 min. to bake

Serves: 4

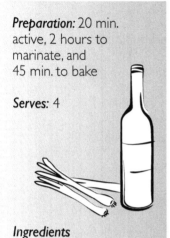

Ingredients

- 1-inch piece fresh ginger
- 1/3 cup balsamic vinegar
- 1/3 cup blackstrap molasses
- 1/4 tsp pepper
- 1½ tsp red miso
- 1 tsp rice wine
- 1/2 tsp turmeric
- 1 Tbs water
- 2 pounds boneless, skinless chicken breasts

- 1 bunch green onions
- 1/3 cup cilantro
- Quinoa or another grain

- 2 cups mixed greens

*M*arinating is a great way to add interest to chicken. If you are a fan of dark meat, go ahead and substitute for the chicken breasts. The molasses marinade gives the chicken a lovely, rich sweetness and a beautiful color. This dish pairs well with cooked grains and mixed greens. Blackstrap molasses is rich in vitamins and minerals, particularly iron, manganese, copper, calcium, potassium, magnesium, vitamin B6, and selenium. Ginger contains powerful anti-inflammatory compounds. Clinical studies have shown that consuming it regularly reduces pain and improves mobility for people with osteoarthritis and rheumatoid arthritis, and growing evidence also supports the antioxidant properties of miso.

Marinade
Grate ginger. In a small pot over medium heat, bring vinegar, molasses, ginger, and pepper to a boil; lower heat and simmer for ten minutes. Combine miso, rice wine, turmeric, and water, and stir into the molasses mixture. Allow to cool. Set half the marinade aside, then refrigerate chicken in remaining marinade for two hours.

Remove chicken from marinade, and discard the used marinade. Preheat oven to 350 degrees.

Prep
Chop green onions and cilantro. Prepare grains according to package directions, enough to make four servings of cooked grains.

Chicken
Bake chicken, covered, in an oiled baking dish for forty-five minutes or until cooked through.

Serve
Serve chicken alongside your favorite grain and mixed greens. Drizzle with remaining unused marinade. Garnish with green onions and cilantro.

Harvest Casserole

Preparation: 20 min.
active, 1 hour to bake

Serves: 4

*T*his lightly sweet autumn casserole is a delicious accompaniment to amaranth.

Pumpkin seeds, also called pepitas, contain a wide variety of antioxidant phytonutrients, and also are a rich source of zinc.

Ingredients

- 3 cups chicken stock
- 1 cup amaranth
- 1 medium winter squash
- 1/2 cup dates
- 2 Tbs almond flour

- 1 tsp salt
- 1 tsp freshly ground pepper
- 1 tsp cinnamon
- 1/2 tsp ground ginger
- 1/2 tsp nutmeg
- 1 tsp turmeric
- 1 Tbs fresh thyme leaves or 1 tsp dried
- 2 Tbs maple syrup
- 1 cup chicken stock
- 1/2 cup coconut cream
- 1/4 cup pumpkin seeds
- 1 Tbs coconut flakes

Prep

In a large saucepan, bring chicken stock to a boil. Add the amaranth, reduce heat, and simmer forty minutes or until the liquid is absorbed.

Preheat oven to 350 degrees. Grease a 9 × 12 baking dish or two-quart casserole.

Peel, seed, and dice the winter squash. Chop dates; toss with almond flour to coat.

Casserole

Place squash and date in baking dish. Combine dry herbs and spices, and sprinkle on top along with fresh thyme, if using.

Combine maple syrup, 1 cup chicken stock, and coconut cream, then pour over ingredients in baking dish.

Bake covered for forty-five minutes. Uncover, sprinkle with pumpkin seeds and coconut flakes, increase heat to 400 degrees, and bake an additional ten minutes.

Serve

Spoon casserole over a bed of amaranth.

Mini-Meatloaf

Preparation: 60 min.

Serves: 4

Ingredients

*M*ini-meatloaf, baked in muffin tins, makes a portable snack, ideal for a picnic or potluck. The individual portions are perfect for making ahead of time and freezing. The sauce includes tomatoes, a nightshade I generally recommend avoiding. But if your body tolerates nightshades in moderation, tomatoes are fantastic antioxidants. You may choose to leave the sauce off entirely. Feel free to substitute seasonally available vegetables of your choice.

Prep
Grate zucchini and carrots. Finely chop onion and kale. Press or mince garlic. Chop thyme, if using fresh.

Preheat oven to 350 degrees. Prepare muffin tins with liners or oil.

- 1 zucchini
- 2 carrots
- 1/3 cup onion
- 1 leaf kale
- 3 cloves garlic
- 2 Tbs fresh thyme or 2 tsp dried

Meatloaf
Heat coconut oil in a large skillet; saute onion, zucchini, and carrot until tender. Add garlic, and saute a few minutes longer; allow to cool slightly.

Combine sauteed ingredients in a large bowl, stir in other ingredients, and mix well. Divide mixture among eight muffin tins, press. Bake for forty-five minutes.

- 2 Tbs coconut oil
- 1½ lbs ground turkey
- 1 large egg
- 1/2 cup almond flour
- 1 tsp Himalayan salt
- 1 tsp cumin
- 1 tsp turmeric
- 1/4 tsp allspice
- 1/4 tsp black pepper

Sauce
Combine ingredients; pour over each mini-meatloaf. Bake an additional fifteen minutes.

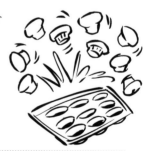

- 3/4 cup tomato sauce
- 1 Tbs coconut sugar
- 1 Tbs blackstrap molasses
- 2 tsp apple cider vinegar
- 1/2 tsp onion powder
- 1/4 tsp Himalayan salt

Serve
Serve mini-meatloaves with additional sauce, if desired.

Moroccan Chicken

Preparation: 20 min. active, 4 or 8 hours in slow cooker

Serves: 4

Ingredients

- Sprouted rice
- 1 onion
- 2 cloves garlic
- 1/2 cup dates
- 2 carrot
- 2 large zucchinis
- 1/4 cup fresh parsley
- 1 inch ginger
- 4 cups chickpeas, soaked overnight (or 2 cans)
- 2 pounds boneless, skinless chicken breast

- 2 Tbs coconut oil

- 2 tsp thyme leaves
- 1 tsp turmeric
- 1/2 tsp cinnamon
- 1/2 tsp pepper
- 1/2 tsp salt
- 1 tsp ground coriander
- 2 bay leaves
- 1½ quarts chicken stock

- 1 cup plain Greek yogurt.

Inspired by the cuisine of Morocco, this chicken is baked in a slow cooker, and is a great dish to come home to on a busy day. In addition to other healing herbs and spices, it includes cinnamon, which has been shown to alleviate factors associated with Alzheimer's disease and ischemic stroke. In addition, growing evidence shows that it decreases inflammation.

Prep
Cook rice according to package directions to make four servings; refrigerate until serving time.

Roughly chop onion, garlic, dates, carrot, zucchini, and parsley. Grate ginger. Rinse and drain chickpeas. Cube chicken.

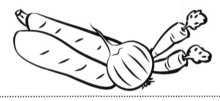

Stovetop
Brown chicken in coconut oil over medium heat. Remove from pan, and place in slow cooker. Saute onion, garlic, and 2 tablespoons chicken stock until onion is translucent, scraping browned bits. Add to slow cooker.

Slow Cooker
Add remaining ingredients (except zucchini and rice) to slow cooker, and cook on low for eight hours or high four hours. Add zucchini in at the last hour.

Serve
Warm rice. Remove bay leaves; serve over rice with a dollop of yogurt.

Roasted Turkey Tenderloin and Vegetables

Preparation: 1 hour, plus 2 hours to marinate.

Serves: 8

Roasting vegetables brings out their natural sweetness which is helpful for introducing cauliflower to the diet. Cauliflower is high in vitamin C, which is best known as an antioxidant, and helps prevent damage to cells. Vitamin C helps to support certain neurotransmitters, an important part of brain health. Mustard, also included in this recipe, is more than simply a condiment; it contains phytonutrients that inhibit cancer cell growth. Furthermore, mustard contains selenium and magnesium, which are powerful anti-inflammatories.

Ingredients

- 3 pounds turkey tenderloin
- 1 cup balsamic vinegar
- 1½ cup extra virgin olive oil
- 3 Tbs Dijon mustard
- 1 Tbs honey

Marinade
Whisk vinegar, oil, mustard, and honey. Marinate turkey in this mixture for 2 hours.

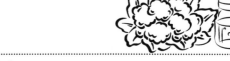

- 2 cloves garlic
- 1 head cauliflower
- 2 sweet potatoes

Prep
Peel and mince garlic. Chop cauliflower into bite-sized pieces. Thinly slice sweet potatoes.
  Preheat oven to 350 degrees.

- 3 Tbs extra virgin olive oil
- 1/2 tsp Himalayan salt
- 1 tsp turmeric

Cauliflower
In a medium bowl, mix oil, salt, turmeric, and garlic. Place cauliflower on a rimmed cookie sheet, drizzle oil mixture over the florets, toss to coat evenly.
  Roast, stirring occasionally, thirty-five to forty-five minutes, until golden brown and tender.

- 4 Tbs fresh basil
- 1/2 tsp salt
- 1/4 tsp pepper

Bake
Put turkey and sweet potatoes in a baking dish; sprinkle with basil, salt, and pepper. Cover and bake fifteen to twenty minutes or until tender.

Serve
Slice turkey and serve with cauliflower and sweet potatoes

Smothered Chicken and Sweet Potatoes

Preparation: 45 min.

Serves: 6

Ingredients

- Quinoa
- 2 pounds boneless skinless chicken
- 1 pound cremini mushrooms
- 1 shallot
- 1 sweet potato

- 2 Tbs coconut oil
- 1 cup chicken broth

- 1 cup coconut milk
- 1 cup chicken broth
- 1 tsp Himalayan salt
- 1 tsp black pepper

- 1 Tbs capers
- 2 cups baby spinach

*T*his is a pretty, warm dish, perfect for entertaining or enjoying at home on a cold day. The sweet potatoes pair beautifully with the mushrooms and the rich coconut milk sauce. There are plenty of healing ingredients, including essential amino acids from the quinoa. Chicken and cremini mushrooms provide B vitamins, particularly B3 (niacin), which is a powerful antioxidant. Spinach provides vitamins A and K, in addition to calcium, magnesium, and zinc. This combination promotes tissue repair and helps to alleviate damage associated with the aging process.

Prep
Preheat oven to 350 degrees.

Cook quinoa according to package directions, enough to make six servings.

Slice chicken into strips. Slice mushrooms. Peel and slice shallot. Dice sweet potato.

Stovetop
In a frying pan, brown chicken in coconut oil on both sides. Add broth, mushrooms, and shallot, and continue to cook a few minutes longer, stirring frequently.

Bake
In a small bowl, whisk coconut milk and another cup of broth.

Place sweet potato in baking dish, add chicken mixture, and sprinkle with salt and pepper. Pour coconut milk and broth over it all. Cover and bake twenty minutes, or until sweet potatoes are soft.

Serve
Just before serving, stir baby spinach into the warm chicken-and-sweet-potato mixture. Spoon over quinoa, and sprinkle with capers.

Stuffed Acorn Squash

Preparation: 15 min.
hands-on, 45 min. baking

Serves: 4

Ingredients

- 1/3 cup toasted pumpkin seeds
- 1 finely chopped shallot
- 3 cups cooked black beans or 2 15-oz. cans, drained and rinsed
- 2 Tbs chopped cilantro
- Quinoa

- 4 acorn squash
- 3 Tbs extra virgin olive oil
- 1 Tbs ground cumin
- 1 tsp ground oregano
- 1/2 tsp salt
- 1/4 cup water or vegetable or chicken stock
- 2 cups chopped fresh spinach
- 1/2 cup crumbled goat or Parmesan cheese

*T*his dish is visually appealing and very nourishing. In addition to antioxidants, each cup of black beans provides fiber and about 15 grams of protein. I've found that the mildly sweet flavor of squash satisfies some of my craving for sweets, while providing vitamin C, beta-carotene, folate, and more fiber. Olive oil has been getting a lot of attention for improving cognitive function, particularly among older adults.

Prep

Preheat oven to 375 degrees.

Toast pumpkin seeds in a dry skillet over medium heat. Peel and finely chop shallot. Drain and rinse black beans. Chop cilantro.

Cook, according to package directions, enough quinoa to make 1½ cups cooked grains.

Cook

Lightly coat large baking sheet with oil or cooking spray. Cut squash in half tip-to-stem. Scoop out and discard seeds. Place squash cut side down on baking sheet. Bake until tender, about forty-five minutes.

Heat olive oil in medium saucepan over medium heat. Add shallot and seasonings. Saute, stirring often, until shallot softens, about five minutes. Stir in water, beans, quinoa, and spinach. Simmer about ten minutes, mashing and stirring mixture with back of a fork. If beans seem too dry, add small amounts of water until desired consistency is reached. Adjust seasonings.

Remove pan from heat. With back of the fork, continue to break up bean mixture to desired consistency.

When squash are tender, remove and reduce oven temperature to 325 degrees. Fill squash halves with bean mixture, and top with cheese. Place on baking sheet, return to oven, and bake until filling is heated through and cheese is melted, 8–10 minutes.

Serve

Garnish squash with cilantro and pumpkin seeds.

Stuffed Sweet Potatoes

Preparation: 20 min. prep plus 1 hour baking

Serves: 4

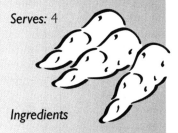

Ingredients

- 4 sweet potatoes
- 4 Tbs coconut oil
- 1 cup walnuts
- 2 diced shallot
- 2 garlic cloves
- 1 can or 2 cups cooked white beans
- 2 bags raw baby spinach
- 1/2 lemon
- 1 tsp cinnamon
- 1/2 tsp nutmeg

- 2 Tbs coconut oil
- 2 sprigs fresh rosemary
- 1/4 cup chicken stock
- Himalayan salt
- freshly ground black pepper
- 3 Tbs coconut oil

- 1 cup shredded coconut
- 1 cup parmesan or goat cheese (optional)

*B*aked sweet potatoes plus healing herbs make a deeply satisfying dinner or lunch. White beans, also known as white navy beans, offer numerous health benefits. They are filled with antioxidants, are a good source of fiber and protein, and rank low on the Glycemic Index. White beans also provide magnesium and are one of the most concentrated food sources of molybdenum and other trace minerals that are extremely important for good health. Molybdenum has detoxifying properties and aids in the metabolism of fats and carbohydrates.

Prep

Preheat oven to 400 degrees.

Coat sweet potatoes with 1 tablespoon of coconut oil. Prick with a fork, and bake, uncovered, for forty-five minutes to an hour.

Finely chop walnuts, and toast them in a dry skillet over medium heat, stirring frequently; set aside. Peel and dice shallot. Peel and mince garlic. Rinse and drain beans. Chop spinach. Juice lemon. In a small dish, combine 3 tablespoons coconut oil, cinnamon, and nutmeg; set aside.

Cook

Start the beans about fifteen to twenty minutes before the sweet potatoes are done. In a large pot or skillet, heat 2 tablespoons coconut oil over medium heat. Add the shallots, and cook until translucent, about five minutes. Add the garlic and rosemary, and cook, stirring, for about a minute. Add the beans and stock, cook for five minutes, stirring occasionally. Add the spinach, cover the pan, and cook, stirring occasionally, for about two minutes, or until the spinach is soft. Remove the rosemary sprigs, stir in the lemon juice, and season to taste with salt and pepper.

Serve

To serve, slice each sweet potato lengthwise and open. Spoon cinnamon mixture on top, and then spoon on the beans. Sprinkle shredded coconut, toasted walnuts, and cheese, if desired, on top.

Dandelion Greens Enchiladas

andelion greens have been used as a traditional medicine in the Middle East at least since the tenth century. They are a great source of fiber and vitamins A and K. Additionally, they protect against Alzheimer's by helping to limit neuron damage in the brain. These enchiladas are a great way to introduce bitter greens into the diet. They have the hearty feel of traditional enchiladas with the added benefits of the greens. If dandelion greens aren't available, feel free to substitute mustard, collard, endive, or another bitter green of your choice. I recommend sprouted grain tortillas, but if they are unavailable, go ahead and use organic corn tortillas. Sprouting grains before use increases digestibility, lowers the starch content, and raises the proportions of protein, vitamins, and minerals.

Preparation: 15 min. prep, 45 min. baking.

Serves: 6

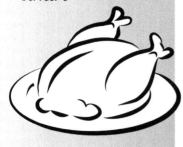

Ingredients

- 1 whole roasted chicken
- 2 bunches green onions
- 1 bunch dandelion greens
- 1/4 pound portabella mushrooms
- 6 cloves garlic

- 2 Tbs olive oil
- 1 cup chicken broth
- 1 package tortillas
- 1 (13-oz) jar green chiles or green chile sauce (including liquid)
- 12 oz shredded organic Mexican cheese

Prep

Debone chicken, tear meat into bite-sized pieces, and set aside. Finely chop green onions, dandelion greens, and mushrooms. Press or mince garlic. Preheat oven to 350 degrees.

Enchiladas

In a soup pot, saute green onions and garlic in olive oil until onions are soft. Add greens and mushrooms, and saute until greens are tender and bright green. Add chicken, broth, and chile. Simmer for ten minutes.

In a 9 x 13 baking dish, layer greens and mushroom mix with cheese and tortillas until dish is full. Bake forty-five minutes, or until cheese is bubbly and begins to brown.

Serve

Serve warm.

Turmeric Chicken and Brussels Sprouts

Preparation: 45 min.

Serves: 4

Ingredients

*Q*uick and easy to prepare, this delicious dish is a great way to introduce brussels sprouts into the diet. Brussels sprouts have many heath benefits, not the least of which is their abundance of vitamin antioxidants, such as vitamins C and beta-carotene, as well as the antioxidant mineral manganese. Brussels sprouts are also powerful anti-inflammatories because of the presence of turmeric, glucosinolates, vitamin K, and Omega-3.

- 1 pound brussels sprouts
- 1 sweet potato
- 4 small shallots
- 1 lemon
- 2 sprigs rosemary
- 2 cloves garlic

- 4 Tbs extra virgin olive oil
- 1 tsp salt
- 1/2 tsp ground pepper
- 1 tsp cumin
- 2 Tbs turmeric
- 1 tsp dried thyme
- 2½ pounds chicken thighs

Prep
Preheat oven to 350 degrees.

Trim and quarter brussels sprouts. Dice sweet potatoes. Peel and quarter shallots. Slice lemon into thin pinwheels. Stem rosemary, and finely chop leaves. Peel and mince garlic.

Bake
Combine brussels sprouts, sweet potato, shallots, lemon, 2 tablespoons oil, 1/4 teaspoon pepper, 1/2 teaspoon salt, and cumin in a large baking dish.

Mash garlic and the remaining 1/2 teaspoon salt with side of a knife to form a paste. Combine with rosemary, turmeric, thyme, remaining 1/4 teaspoon pepper, and remaining 2 tablespoon oil. Rub paste over chicken. Nestle chicken in with brussels sprouts and sweet potato.

Roast, lightly covered with foil, until done, about twenty minutes for bone-in, and ten to twelve minutes for boneless.

Serve
Serve chicken with brussels sprouts and sweet potato.

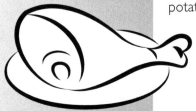

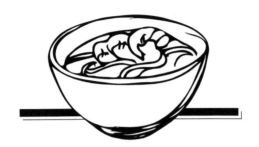

Meat, Poultry, and Fish Entrees

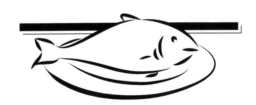

Glazed Chicken Skewers

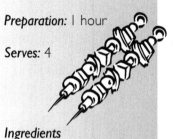

Preparation: 1 hour

Serves: 4

Ingredients

These delicious skewers are the perfect grilling-weather treat. If it's too blustery to cook outside, go ahead and broil them on a cookie sheet in the oven. Chia seeds are high in Omega-3 fats and fiber, as well as protein and manganese. Healing herbs such as cinnamon and nutmeg are anti-inflammatories and offer additional brain support. Animal studies also have shown promising results from using cinnamon in the treatment of cognitive decline.

- 1 large sweet potato
- 2 cups quinoa

On the stove
Peel sweet potato, cut into sixteen pieces. In a saucepan with a steamer basket, bring 1 inch of water to a boil over high heat. Steam the sweet potato until nearly cooked but still a bit firm, ten to twelve minutes. Remove from heat; set aside.
Cook quinoa according to package instructions.

- 1 cup sherry vinegar
- 1/2 cup plus 1 Tbs honey
- 2 Tbs coconut oil
- Himalayan salt to taste
- Black pepper to taste

Glaze
In small saucepan, add vinegar, ½ cup honey, 1 tablespoon oil, salt, and pepper. Simmer over medium heat, stirring occasionally until reduced to 2/3 cup, thirteen to fifteen minutes.

- 1 pound boneless, skinless chicken breast halves
- 4 spring onions

Prepare Skewers
Cut chicken and onions into sixteen pieces. Thread onions, chicken, and sweet potatoes onto the skewers. Use half the glaze to brush the skewers. Oil the grill; arrange the skewers on half of the grill; turn as necessary.

- 1/2 cup walnuts
- 1 tsp cumin
- 1 tsp cinnamon
- 1/2 tsp ground nutmeg
- 1/2 tsp ground ginger
- 1 Tbs chia seeds

Topping
Chop the walnuts coarsely, then toss them in a small bowl with the remaining honey and oil. Add cumin, cinnamon, nutmeg, ginger, chia seeds, salt, and a pinch of pepper. Grill nuts on foil on the other half of the grill. Cook until the chicken is cooked through and the nuts are sizzling, three to five minutes.

Serve
Brush skewers with remaining glaze, and sprinkle with walnuts. Serve on a bed of quinoa.

Garlic Shrimp with Kale

Preparation: 30 min.

Serves: 4

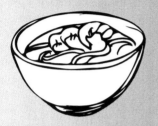

Ingredients

- 1 pound raw shrimp
- 3 tsp garlic
- 2 Tbs ginger
- 1 bunch kale
- 2 lemons

- 2 cups polenta cornmeal
- 6 cups water
- 1/2 tsp salt

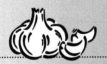

- 1 Tbs coconut oil
- 2 Tbs red wine vinegar
- 1 Tbs turmeric
- 1/2 tsp salt
- 1/4 tsp pepper

- 1/4 cup parmesan

I *don't recommend eating corn or corn products often, but occasionally, a polenta dish like this one hits all the right notes. This dish is visually pleasing, as well as offering a range of flavors and textures that are sure to please even the most reluctant eaters. Corn has been domesticated for over 10,000 years. It is a rich source of antioxidant phytonutrients, and the process of drying corn into cornmeal for polenta does not significantly alter its antioxidant properties. Corn is a good source of fiber, and offers digestive and blood sugar benefits. In addition to its powerful anti-inflammatory components, ginger has a long history of alleviating symptoms of gastrointestinal distress.*

Prep
Peel and de-vein shrimp. Thinly slice garlic. Grate ginger. Separate kale leaves from stems, thinly slice stems and cut leaves into ribbons. Slice lemons.

Polenta
Bring water to boil and add salt. Reduce heat to medium-low, sprinkle 1/3 of the polenta into the pot. Stir constantly for about two minutes, add the remaining polenta to the pot, keep stirring for a further 10 minutes. Polenta should be creamy but not mushy. Remove from heat when it reaches the consistency you like.

Shrimp
Saute garlic, ginger and turmeric in coconut oil over medium heat. Add shrimp and continue to cook, stirring frequently, until opaque. Add kale and vinegar, reduce heat to low. Cook until kale wilts, stir in salt and pepper.

Serve
Divide polenta among bowls, add shrimp and kale mixture. Sprinkle with parmesan, and garnish with a slice or two of lemon.

Pan-Fried Tilapia

Preparation: 15 min.

Serves: 2

Ingredients

- 1 pound shiitake mushrooms
- 3 limes
- 2 shallots
- 2 cloves garlic
- 1 cup cilantro
- 2 tsp salt
- 4 tilapia fillets

- 3 Tbs coconut oil
- 2 tsp chile powder
- 1 tsp pepper

- 4 cups mixed baby greens

*H*ealing mushrooms and spices really jazz up tilapia's gentle flavor. This dish cooks up fairly quickly, and is great for a filling yet light meal. Mushrooms have many health benefits, including supporting the immune system and protection against cardiovascular disease. The Chinese have long revered shiitake mushrooms for their medicinal properties. They are a strong source of iron, and are rich in B vitamins, which have been shown to support brain health. Additionally, they contain an abundant amount of manganese, selenium, copper, and zinc.

Prep

Prep mushrooms by wiping clean and slicing thinly. Juice two limes, and slice the other into wedges. Peel and thinly slice shallot. Peel and press or mince garlic. Roughly chop cilantro.

Mix salt and lime juice; pour over tilapia.

Fish

In a skillet, heat coconut oil, and cook fish over medium heat two to three minutes on each side. Remove from pan and set aside.

Add shiitake mushrooms, shallot, salt, pepper, garlic, and chile powder to skillet. Cook for another two or three minutes, or until mushrooms are soft.

Serve

Divide fillets among dishes; top with mushrooms. Serve on a bed of mixed baby greens. Garnish with a slice of lime and cilantro.

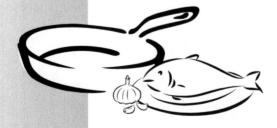

Salmon With Lemon Relish

Preparation: 15 min. active plus 1 hour to bake

Serves: 4

Ingredients

- 1 medium shallot, minced
- 1 Tbs champagne vinegar
- 1/2 tsp Himalayan salt
- 2 lemons
- sprouted brown rice

- 1/4 cup olive oil
- 2 Tbs chopped cilantro
- 1/4 tsp freshly ground pepper

- 2 pounds salmon filet
- 1/4 cup olive oil
- 1 tsp Himalayan salt
- 1 tsp freshly ground pepper

- 4 cups mixed greens

*T*his is a lovely way to prepare salmon; the pan of water creates a moist environment, and the low baking temperature allows the salmon to cook slowly, virtually ensuring success. The lemon relish is a tasty complement to salmon's natural sweetness. Salmon is prized for its high levels of Omega-3 fatty acids, but it has many other benefits as well, including bioactive peptides that provide support for joint cartilage, insulin effectiveness, and control of inflammation in the digestive tract. Salmon also is rich in vitamins B3, B6, and D and the minerals selenium and phosphorus, as well as protein.

Prep

Peel and mince shallot, mix with vinegar and salt, set aside. Slice lemons into sixteenths, and remove core and seeds. Slice wedges into very thin triangles.

Make sprouted brown rice according to package directions, enough for four servings.

Preheat oven to 200 degrees.

Salmon

Add lemons, olive oil, cilantro, and pepper to the shallot mixture. Mix well, and refrigerate until salmon is done.

Relish

Place a baking dish with water in the lowest rack of the oven. Rub salmon with oil, and sprinkle with salt and pepper. Place on a baking sheet and bake, uncovered, forty-five minutes to an hour, or until the fish is firm to the touch and juices start to bead on the surface.

Serve

Serve salmon on a bed of mixed greens, with a side of sprouted brown rice and a heaping spoonful of relish.

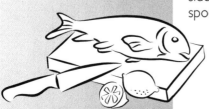

Steak With Ginger Marinade

Preparation: 20 min., plus
4 hours to marinate.

Serves: 4

K ale on the grill! Who would have thought? This is an impressive and easy meal, though you do need to plan for marinating time. Fresh ginger root is available year-round, and is well worth choosing over dried ginger. It is native to southeastern Asia, where it has been used since ancient times. Popular the world over, it is now grown in many other tropical regions. Ginger offers many benefits, including gastrointestinal support and anti-inflammatory and cancer protection, in addition to boosting immunity.

Ingredients

- 2 inches fresh ginger
- 3 cloves garlic
- 3 limes
- 2 bunches kale
- 3 Tbs cilantro

Prep
Peel and grate ginger. Juice limes. Cut stems from kale leaves, leaving leaves whole. Finely chop cilantro.

- 1 ½ pounds steak
- 1/2 tsp black pepper
- 1 tsp turmeric

Meat Marinade
Stir ginger, garlic, pepper, turmeric, cilantro, and 4 tablespoons lime juice. Coat steak with this mixture. Marinate, covered, in refrigerator at least 4 hours, flipping occasionally.

- 2 cans coconut milk
- 2 Tbs tamari

Kale Marinade
In a small bowl, whisk together coconut milk, tamari, and remaining lime juice. Pour over kale and marinate, covered, in refrigerator, at least 4 hours.

Grill
Grill kale leaves over high heat, one to two minutes per side. Cut into smaller pieces to serve.

Grill steak four to five minutes per side for rare, or six to eight minutes per side for well done. Let sit for a few minutes, and slice.

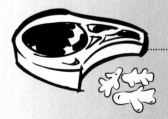

Serve
Divide kale among plates, topped with steak.

Tilapia With Pesto

Preparation: 45 min.

Serves: 4

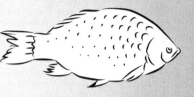

Ingredients

- 4 cloves garlic
- 2 leafs chard
- 1½-inch piece of ginger
- 1 lemon

- 2 Tbs butter
- 4 fillets tilapia
- 1/4 tsp salt

- 1/2 cup coconut milk
- 3 cups fresh basil leaves, tightly packed
- 4 oz. mixed sprouts
- 1/3 cup unsweetened shredded coconut
- 1/4 cup extra virgin olive oil
- 1/4 cup cashews
- 1 Tbs plum vinegar
- a few sprigs fresh mint

*H*omemade pesto is a refreshing summertime pleasure. You can find potted basil plants at many groceries throughout the summer, and they are even cheaper than buying harvested basil leaves. Basil is related to peppermint, and has many health benefits. It is recognized as an anti-inflammatory food that helps for many conditions ranging from rheumatoid arthritis to Alzheimer's disease. Tilapia, a mild, white fish, is a great "starter" fish for those who are unaccustomed to seafood. Because the tilapia fish eats plants, it is one of the safer seafood choices in terms of mercury. It is also inexpensive and readily available.

Prep
Mince or press 2 cloves of the garlic, and roughly chop 2 more cloves. Roughly chop chard, including stem. Grate ginger. Juice lemon.
Preheat oven to 375 degrees. Grease a 9 x 13 baking dish.

Fish
Melt butter, stir in 2 cloves garlic and salt. Pour butter mixture over tilapia in baking dish. Cover and bake twenty-five minutes, or until fish flakes easily with a fork.

Pesto
While fish is baking, combine remainder of garlic, chard, ginger, lemon juice, coconut milk, basil, sprouts, shredded coconut, olive oil, cashews, vinegar, and mint in a blender; process until desired consistency is reached. Add more coconut milk if mixture is too thick to pulse.

Serve
When fish is done, allow to cool slightly, and serve with pesto.

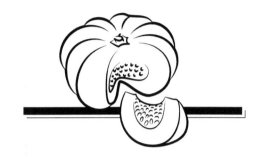

Vegetarian Entrees

Burdock Root Delight

Preparation: 45 min.

Serves: 4

Ingredients

- 2 cups burdock
- 1 carrot
- 1 sweet potato
- 2 cups broccoli
- 2 cups kale

- 2 Tbs coconut oil
- 4 cups chicken broth
- 1/4 cup tamari

*R*elated to the dandelion, burdock root provides a base for this delightfully simple, unpretentious dish. Pretty and flavorful, it is sure to impress even the most die-hard meat fans in your life. Though burdock root has been prized for its healing properties in traditional Asian and European societies for centuries, Western medicine is just beginning to recognize its potential as an anti-inflammatory, antioxidant, and antibacterial agent. Burdock is rich in calcium, flavonoids, iron, and potassium, which is an important component of cell and body fluids that help control heart rate and blood pressure.

Prep
Peel and slice burdock root; julienne carrot. Dice sweet potato. Chop up broccoli and kale.

Cook
Heat oil in large pot; add burdock, carrot, sweet potato, and chicken broth. Bring to a boil, reduce heat, and simmer covered for twenty minutes.

Add broccoli and kale, and return to a boil; cover and simmer five minutes more. Remove from heat, and stir in tamari.

Serve
Ladle into bowls and enjoy!

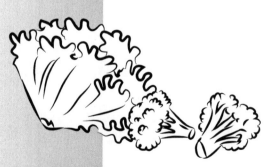

Herbed Brown Rice Medley

Preparation: 45 min.

Serves: 4

*T*his is a complex, interesting dish. Visually stunning, it also provides a wealth of textures and health benefits. Brown rice is rich in manganese, which is a powerful antioxidant. Manganese also helps in the synthesis of fatty acids, which are critical for a healthy nervous system. For those who are avoiding grains, feel free to substitute roasted sweet potato or a winter squash of your choice. Pumpkin seeds are a fantastic source of zinc, which supports immune function and skin health.

Ingredients

- I cup brown rice
- I ½ cups vegetable broth
- 1/4 cup pumpkin seeds
- 1/3 cup cilantro
- I cup spinach
- I clove garlic
- 1/2 cup celery
- 1/2 lemon

- 3 Tbs extra virgin olive oil
- I Tbs walnut oil
- 1/2 tsp salt
- 1/2 tsp ground pepper
- 1/4 feta cheese
- 1/2 dried cranberries

Prep
Cook rice in a medium saucepan with broth, according to package instructions. Allow to cool.

Toast pumpkin seeds in a dry skillet over medium heat, stirring occasionally.

Finely chop cilantro, spinach, and garlic. Slice celery and lemon.

Assemble
In a small bowl, combine oils, salt, and pepper; whisk gently. In a large bowl, combine cilantro, spinach, and garlic. Toss with oil mixture. Stir in celery, salt, pepper, pumpkin seeds, and rice. Sprinkle with feta and cranberries. Toss again right before serving.

Serve
Serve with a squeeze of lemon.

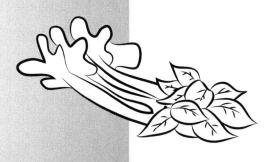

Nori Wraps

Preparation: 30 min.

Serves: 4

Ingredients

- Sprouted rice
- 1 daikon radish
- 1/2 tsp salt
- 3 Tbs tamari
- 2 tsp ginger
- 1 carrot
- 1 cucumber
- 1 avocado

- 4 dried nori seaweed sheets

*N*ori wraps look complicated but are actually quite easy. While there is a bit of a technique to the rolling—and it's true that traditional, authentic technique requires years of study—you can create a delicious echo of the real thing in your own kitchen. Nori is edible seaweed that comes in sheets and is readily available in the U.S. It is a dark purple-black in color that turns phosphorescent green when toasted. Sea vegetables are an excellent source of bioavailable iron and vitamin C, and also are also a unique food source of the minerals iodine and vanadium.

Prep
Cook sprouted rice according to package directions, enough to make 2 cups cooked rice.
  Finely chop radish, enough to make 1 cup. Add to food processor, along with rice, salt, and tamari, and pulse until minced. Grate ginger, and stir into rice mixture. Slice carrot and cucumber into fine slivers. Peel and cube avocado.

Roll
Toast nori sheets over an open flame quickly to just give them a bright green sheen. Place one sheet on a towel; spread rice to three edges, leaving 1 inch of the fourth edge bare to close the roll. Place a quarter of the veggies along the bottom of the rice and roll, using the towel to help maintain pressure. Seal the roll with a small amount of water.

Serve
Slice rolls, and offer more tamari for dipping.

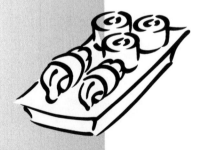

Quinoa Bean Bowl

Preparation: 20 min.

Serves: 4

Ingredients

- 1 cup quinoa
- 2 cups chicken or vegetable broth
- 2 green onions
- 2 cloves minced garlic
- 1/4 head cabbage, shredded
- 2 (15-oz.) cans black beans
- 1 avocado
- 2 limes
- 1/4 cup cilantro

- 1 Tbs coconut oil
- 1/4 tsp chili powder
- 1½ tsp cumin
- 1/2 cup goat cheese crumbles (optional)

*T*his delicious dish makes a hearty lunch. Cabbage has a long history of use as both a food and a medicine. It is a cruciferous vegetable, rich in antioxidants, and is prized for its anti-inflammatory properties, which can slow the progression of cognitive decline. Cabbage is also an excellent source of vitamins B6, C, and K and a very good source of manganese, potassium, and dietary fiber. Stirring the cabbage in at the last minute is a good way to avoid overcooking it. You also may want to sprinkle goat cheese on top.

Prep
Cook quinoa in broth according to package directions. Chop green onions. Press or mince garlic. Shred cabbage. Drain and rinse beans.

Peel and cube avocado. Juice limes. Chop cilantro. In a small bowl, toss avocado, lime juice, and cilantro; set aside.

Cook
In a deep skillet, saute onions and garlic in coconut oil. Add chili powder, cumin, and black beans. Continue to heat until black beans are warm. Stir in cabbage and quinoa, and cook a few minutes longer.

Serve
Divide among bowls; garnish with avocado mixture.

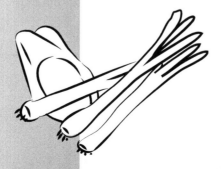

Quinoa Pilaf

Preparation: 30 min.

Serves: 4

Ingredients

- 1/2 cup quinoa
- 1/4 cup pumpkin seeds
- 1 large shallot
- 1½ cups zucchini

- 3 cups vegetable or chicken broth or water
- 2 Tbs extra-virgin olive oil
- 1/2 tsp ground ginger
- 1/2 cup crumbled goat cheese
- salt to taste

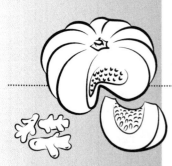

*Q*uinoa is a versatile grain and easy to prepare. Recently rediscovered, this ancient cereal is thought to have been the "gold of the Incas," and is one of the least allergenic of all grains. It is high in protein, includes all the essential amino acids, and is an excellent source of fiber and a very good source of iron and magnesium. Quinoa is excellent for cognitive support, as it is high in vitamin B12, which supports brain cells, and manganese, an antioxidant. This quinoa pilaf can be a side or a main dish. And you can add chicken and/or substitute a variety of vegetables—such as spinach, chard, artichokes, or carrots—for the zucchini.

Prep
Preheat oven to 350 degrees.

In a fine sieve, rinse quinoa under cold running water for one to two minutes to remove its coating of saponin, a bitter, resin-like glucoside. Set aside.

On an ungreased baking sheet, arrange pumpkin seeds in a layer and bake for three to five minutes, or until slightly darkened. Set aside.

Peel and chop shallot. Chop zucchini.

Pilaf
Add quinoa and broth or water to saucepan, bring to boil, then reduce heat to maintain a gentle simmer. Cover and cook until quinoa is tender and most of the liquid has been absorbed (twenty to twenty-five minutes).

Meanwhile, in saucepan, heat oil over medium heat. Add shallot and ginger, and saute, stirring often, until softened (three to five minutes). Add zucchini and stir until tender (five to seven minutes).

When quinoa is cooked, add shallot and zucchini mixture, and mix in goat cheese. Stir to fluff; add salt to taste.

Serve
Serve hot, topped with toasted pumpkin seeds.

Spaghetti Squash and Ruby Red Beet Sauce

Preparation: 1 hour

Serves: 4

*B*eets make a surprisingly delicious red sauce that pairs beautifully with spaghetti squash. This is a winter squash that has long, tender, noodle-like flesh which makes a fun alternative to pasta. Winter squash are prized for their abundant B vitamins, including B1, B3, B6, pantothenic acid, and folate, and their carotenoid content provides antioxidant benefits. Winter squash also contains moderate amounts of Omega-3 fats in the form of alpha-linolenic acid, which plays a role in supporting cognitive function.

Ingredients

- 1 spaghetti squash
- 1 Tbs coconut oil
- 1 medium shallot
- 4 cloves garlic
- 2 medium beets
- 1/2 cup cauliflower
- 2 carrots
- 1/2 cup fresh basil

- 1 Tbs coconut oil
- 1 Tbs fresh thyme
- 1 Tbs fresh rosemary
- 1½ cups vegetable broth
- 1/2 cup coconut milk
- 1 tsp Himalayan salt

Prep

Preheat oven to 350 degrees.

Cut spaghetti squash lengthwise, scoop out seeds, and spread coconut oil over cut sides. Place squash cut sides down in a baking dish, and bake forty-five minutes or until tender.

Peel and chop shallot, garlic, beets, and cauliflower. Chop carrots and basil.

Sauce

Heat coconut oil in a large, heavy pot over medium heat. Add shallot and garlic, and cook until shallot is translucent, stirring frequently. Add beets, carrots, thyme, and rosemary, and cook for a few more minutes.

Add 1/2 cup broth, coconut milk, and salt; bring to a boil. Reduce heat, cover, and simmer for thirty minutes, stirring occasionally.

Remove from heat; use an immersion blender or carefully transfer to a countertop blender, and puree along with 1 cup broth. Return to pot, add basil, and warm for a few more minutes.

Serve

When squash is done, scoop out the flesh, and fluff with a fork. Divide among plates, and drizzle with sauce.

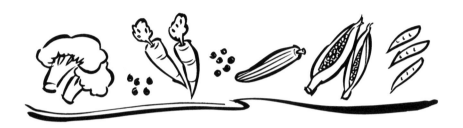

Sample One-Week Menu

Day	Breakfast	Lunch	Dinner
Sunday	Pumpkin Pancakes	Mini Meatloaf	Glazed Chicken Skewers
Monday	Breakfast Burrito	Avocado and Watercress Salad	Beef Stir-Fry
Tuesday	Granola and Goat Yogurt	Kale and Beet Salad	Black Bean and Sweet Potato Soup
Wednesday	Egg Cups	Curried Vegetable Saute	Golden Chicken
Thursday	Quinoa Bean Bowl	Broccoli and Almond Soup	Garlic Shrimp and Kale
Friday	Spinach Mushroom Frittata	Beet and Yogurt Salad	Pan-Fried Tilapia
Saturday	Amaranth Pancakes	Ginger Turkey Cutlets	Dandelion Greens Enchiladas

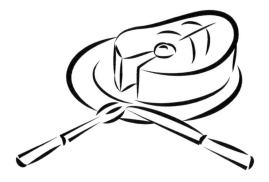

Acknowledgments

This book would not have been possible without the many contributions from my community of family and friends. I would like to thank Ismael for his support of this project over the past three years in all the subtle and behind-the-scenes ways he showed up for me. For my children, Madeleine and Gracie, who tried recipes and offered feedback, courageously sampling new foods outside of their comfort zones.

Thank you to Jessica, who, from the beginning, offered her unwavering support, wisdom, and guidance. Thank you Darrel for his thoughtful critique, helping me strive always to make recipes that are worth "crossing the road for." Thanks to Marilynn for her openness to trying food choices outside her experience. Thanks to Peg who was instrumental in our test kitchen, cooking out the recipes week after week with patience and enthusiasm, and to her son Hawk who enthusiastically added his voice to my own children's taste-testing.

Much gratitude to Chrissy, who helped distill my thoughts and capture the essence of my vision. To Ann, who offered steadfast moral support and optimism. To Tom for his expertise, insights, and guidance on the recipes. To Jody, who encouraged me in the homestretch of this process. And finally, many thanks to my friends who believed in me and held my vision when I lost my way: Emma, Terri, Deborah, Elisa, Karan and Pam, my sweet Mom's Circle (Harmony, Cameron, Elizabeth, Karen, and Audrey), and to the Ya Yas (Patti, Kate, Sandi, and Vicki) for their lifetime of support and belief in me.

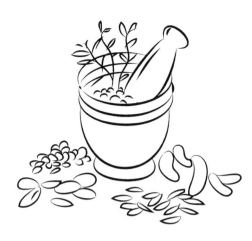

Glossary: Understanding Health and Nutrition

Antioxidant   A molecule that prevents or delays cell damage caused by free radicals.

Atrophy   Shrinkage of cells, reducing their functioning. Although this is a normal part of aging, the rate is much faster in Alzheimer's patients.

Carbohydrates   Organic compounds occurring in food which are broken down to release energy for the body. Carbohydrates come in simple forms, which are sugars, and complex forms, like starches and fiber.

Flavonoids   A family of nutrients with antioxidant and anti-inflammatory properties. Some foods high in flavonoids are parsley, onions, blueberries, and black tea.

Free Radicals   A kind of molecule that causes oxidative damage to the body if it is not neutralized by antioxidants.

Glucose	Sugar in the blood.
Glycemic Index (G.I.)	A measure of the extent to which carbohydrate-containing foods raise the sugar level in your blood, which could increase the risk of diabetes and other diseases.
Glycemic Load	A measure of the carbohydrates in a food, and thus how much the food will raise the blood glucose level when consumed.
Good Fats	Those that are healthy for the body, particularly in preserving brain function. Foods that contain them include fish like salmon, mackerel, and herring, avocados, and cheese. A major category of good fats is the Omega-3 fatty acids.
High Glycemic Foods	Those with a G.I. of 70 or more, which can cause a highly undesirable rapid increase in blood glucose. Examples of these foods are white bread, corn flakes, puffed rice, potatoes, and popcorn.
High Glycemic Load	Foods with a glycemic load of 20 or more. These include high-sugar beverages, sweetened fruit juices, and candy.
Highly Processed Carbohydrates	Those that have been refined or altered in other ways to make them more easily digested, able to last longer, or for other reasons. This can remove healthy components in addition to increasing the food's calories. Many people consume sugars and other processed carbohydrates in white bread, pastries, and soda.
Inflammation	A reaction of the body to injury or infection. Acute inflammation after injury is a normal part of healing. Chronic inflammation, on the other hand, is longer lasting and increases the risk of developing dementia as well as conditions such as cardiovascular disease, diabetes, and cancer. Inflammation impairs the healthy functioning of our organs and bodily systems.
Inflammatory Load	A measure of the markers for inflammation found in blood or other tissues. A high inflammatory load raises the risk of developing a range of chronic conditions.

Inflammatory Markers	Proteins and other kinds of cells that are measured in blood plasma to give information about inflammation and the body's response to it.
Insulin	A hormone made by the pancreas that keeps the level of glucose (sugar) in the blood from getting too high or too low.
Insulin Resistance	A condition in which the body's responsiveness to insulin is reduced.
Ketones	Chemicals the body produces when it uses fats rather than glucose for energy. A high amount of ketones in the blood or urine may mean the body is not producing enough insulin.
Low Glycemic Foods	Those with a G.I. of 55 or less, which raise blood sugar more slowly than medium and high glycemic foods, reducing the risk of dementia and many other chronic conditions. These foods include dried beans and legumes, non-starchy vegetables, sweet potatoes, most fruit, and many whole grain breads and cereals.
Macronutrients	Those that the body requires in large amounts in the diet, such as protein, carbohydrates, and fat.
Metabolism	The body's process for changing nutrients into the form it uses for energy, growth, healing, and the other processes of life.
Micronutrients	Those that the body needs in only small amounts.
Mild Cognitive Impairment	The level of mental decline between what is normal for a person's age and the more serious decline of dementia. It can involve problems with memory, language, thinking, and/or judgment.
Mitochondria	The part of a cell in which energy is created.
Neurodegenerative	Impairing the functioning of brain cells.

Nightshades The plant family (Solanaceae) that includes tomatoes, eggplant, many peppers, potatoes, and tobacco.

Nutrients Compounds in foods that the body uses to survive and grow.

Nutrient-Dense Foods Those with high amounts of nutrients relative to their calories. These include fruits, vegetables, whole grains, seafood, lean poultry and meats, beans, eggs, and unsalted nuts.

Omega-3 Fatty Acids An essential type of fat for the body. Main food sources for this are salmon, mackerel, sardines, and crustaceans.

Omega-6 Fatty Acids A type of fat that is essential in small amount but causes inflammation in larger amounts. It is found in most vegetable oils such as corn oil, safflower oil, and soybean oil, as well as poultry and eggs.

Oxidation Part of the process by which the body produces energy through metabolism. A byproduct of oxidation known as free radicals can damage body cells if antioxidants in the system do not neutralize them.

Oxidative Stress The damage caused by free radicals that are not neutralized by antioxidants. This damage leads to aging, and is a characteristic of Alzheimer's disease.

Phytochemicals Also known as phytonutrients, these compounds give plants characteristics such as smell and color, and also can protect against disease, although the body does not get nutrition from them.

Polyphenol A type of antioxidant that protects cells against the damage caused by free radicals. Research suggests that polyphenols can prevent or limit the effects of dementia and other age-related disorders. They are found in many fruits, berries, grapes, vegetables, walnuts, and tea leaves.

Polyunsaturated Fatty Acids	A type of fat found in nuts, seeds, fish, and leafy greens that has been associated with a reduced risk of dementia. Omega-3 is a polyunsaturated fat.
Processed Food	Any food that has been altered from its natural state, usually for reasons of safety or convenience. Nutrients are often lost when this is done, and salt, sugar, and fat are added.
Recommended Daily Allowance (R.D.A.)	The amount of nutrients and calories that leading scientific bodies consider necessary to maintain good health.
Simple Carbohydrates	Composed of sugars, these are the quickest source of energy because they are digested very rapidly.
Superfoods	A marketing term given to foods said to reduce chronic disease because they contain large amounts of antioxidants, vitamins, and minerals. Chia and blueberries are considered "superfoods."
Whole Foods	Those that have been processed or refined as little as possible and are free from additives or other artificial substances.

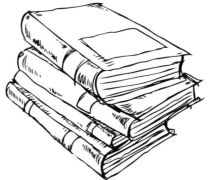

Bibliography

Abuznait AH, Qosa H, Busnena B, El Sayed KA, and Kaddoumi A. "Olive-Oil-Derived Oleocanthal Enhances ß-Amyloid Clearance as a Potential Neuroprotective Mechanism Against Alzheimer's Disease: In Vitro and in Vivo Studies." *ACS Chemical Neuroscience* 4.6 (2013): 973-982.

Akiyama H, Barger S, Barnum S, Bradt B, Bauer J, Cole GM, Cooper NR, Eikelenboom P, Emmerling M, Fiebich BL, Finch CE, Frautschy S, Griffin WS, Hampel H, Hull M, Landreth G, Lue L, Mrak R, Mackenzie IR, McGeer PL, O'Banion MK, Pachter J, Pasinetti G, Plata-Salaman C, Rogers J, Rydel R, Shen Y, Streit W, Strohmeyer R, Tooyoma I, Van Muiswinkel FL, Veerhuis R, Walker D, Webster S, Wegrzyniak B, Wenk G, and Wyss-Coray T. "Inflammation and Alzheimer's Disease." *Neurobiology of Aging* 21.3 (2000): 383-421.

Alzheimer's Organization. *Alzheimer's Facts and Figures. 2013.* 16 July 2013 http://www.alz.org/alzheimers_disease_ facts_and_figures.asp. Amor S, Puentes F, Baker D, and Van Der Valk P. "Inflammation in Neurodegenerative Diseases." *Immunology* 129 (2010): 154–169.

Anand P, Kunnumakkara AB, Newman RA, and Aggarwal BB. "Bioavailability of Curcumin: Problems and Promises." *Molecular Pharmaceutics* 4.6 (2007): 807-818.

Basnet P(1) and Skalko-Basnet N. "Curcumin: An Anti-Inflammatory Molecule From a Curry Spice on the Path to Cancer Treatment." *Molecules.* 3:16(6) (2011): 4567-4598. doi: 10.3390/molecules16064567.

Blennow K, de Leon MJ, and Zetterberg H. "Alzheimer's Disease." *Lancet* 2006; 368-387.

Bredesen DE. "Reversal of Cognitive Decline: A Novel Therapeutic Program." *Aging* 6.9 (n.d.): 707-717.

Butterfield D, Castegna A, Pocernich C, Drake J, Scapagnini G, and Calabrese V. "Nutritional Approaches to Combat Oxidative Stress in Alzheimer's Disease." *The Journal of Nutritional Biochemistry* 13.8 (2002): 444-461.

Chandra V, Pandav R, Dodge HH, Johnston JM, Belle SH, DeKosky ST, and Ganguli M. "Incidence of Alzheimer's Disease in a Rural Community in India: The Indo-US Study." *Neurology* 57.6 (2001): 985-989.

Childress, NF. "A Relationship of Arthritis to the Solanaceae (Nightshades)." *Journal of the International Academy of Preventive Medicine* (1982): 31-37.

Costantini LC, Vogel JL, Barr LJ, Henderson ST. "Clinical Efficacy of AC-1202 (Ketasyn™) in Mild to Moderate Alzheimer's Disease." Paper presented at the 59th annual meeting of the American Academy of Neurology, "Late-Breaking Science" Session, Boston, MA (2007).

Cornutiu G. "The Epidemiological Scale of Alzheimer's Disease." *Journal of Clinical Medicine Research* 7.9 (2015): 657–666.

Corrada MM., et al. "Reduced Risk of Alzheimer's Disease With High Folate Intake: The Baltimore Longitudinal Study of Aging." *Alzheimer's & Dementia: The Journal of the Alzheimer's Association* 1.1 (n.d.): 11-18.

Devere R. "Ketones—A New Treatment for Alzheimer's Disease?" *Practical Neurology*, 14-16. www.practicalneurology.org/issues/0509/PN0509_07.php.

Douaud G, et al. "Preventing Alzheimer's Disease-Related Gray Matter Atrophy by B-Vitamin Treatment." *PNAS* 110.23 (2013): 9523–9528.

Enig MO. "Coconut Oil Is Highly Effective Against Inflammation and Is Also Rich in the Antimicrobial Fatty Acid, Lauric Acid. *Know Your Fats.* Bethesda, MD: Bethesda Press; 2000.

Farr SA, Price TO, Dominguez LJ, Motisi A, Saiano F, Niehoff ML, Morley JE, Banks WA, Ercal N, and Barbagallo M. "Extra Virgin Olive Oil Improves Learning and Memory in SAMP8 Mice." *Journal of Alzheimer's Disease* 28.1 (2012): 81-92.

Feart C, et al. "Adherence to a Mediterranean Diet, Cognitive Decline, and Risk of Dementia." *JAMA* 302.6 (2009).

Frydman-Marom A, Levin A, Farfara D, Benromano T, Scherzer-Attali R, Peled S, Vassar R, Segal D, Gazit E, Frenkel D, and Ovadia M. "Orally Administered Cinnamon Extract Reduces ß-Amyloid Oligomerization and Corrects Cognitive Impairment in Alzheimer's Disease Animal Models." *PLoS One.* 28 January 2011. Ed. Johns Hopkins, United States of America Ted Dawson. 17 July 2013

Grossi C, Rigacci S, Ambrosini S, Ed Dami T, Luccarini I, Traini C, Failli P, Berti A, Casamenti F, and Stefani M. "The Polyphenol Oleuropein Aglycone Protects TgCRND8 Mice Against Aß Plaque Pathology ." *PLoS* (2013).

Hafner-Bratkovi I, Gašperši J, Šmid LM, Bresjanac M, and Jerala R. "Curcumin Binds to the Alpha-Helical Intermediate and to the Amyloid Form of Prion Protein—A New Mechanism for the Inhibition of PrPsc Accumulation." *Journal of Neurochemistry* 104 (2008): 1553–1564.

Henderson ST, Vogel JL, Barr LJ, Garvin F, Jones JJ, Costantini LC. "Study of the Ketogenic Agent AC-1202 in Mild to Moderate Alzheimer's Disease: A Randomized, Double-Blind, Placebo-Controlled, Multicenter Trial." *Nutr Metab* (Lond), vol. 6, no.31, pp.1619-1644, 2009.

Keto-dementia Diet, www.centerwatch.com

Krikorian R, Shidler MD, Dangelo K, Couch SC, Benoit SC, and Clegg DJ. "Dietary ketosis enhances memory in mild cognitive impairment." *Neurobiol Aging* 33:2 (2012): 425-427. Epub 2012.

Lim GP, Chu T, Yang F, Beech W, Frautschy SA, and Cole GM. "The Curry Spice Curcumin Reduces Oxidative Damage and Amyloid Pathology in an Alzheimer Transgenic Mouse." *J Neurosci* (2001) 1;21(21):8370-8377.

Lin C, Yu K, Jheng C, Chung R, and Lee C. "Curcumin Reduces Amyloid Fibrillation of Prion Protein and Decreases Reactive Oxidative Stress." *Pathogens 2* (2013): 506-519.

Mathuranath PS, et al. "Incidence of Alzheimer's Disease in India: A 10 Years Follow-up Study." *Neurology India* 60.6 (2012): 625–630.

Mishra S and Palanivelu K. "The Effect of Curcumin (Turmeric) on Alzheimer's Disease: An Overview. January 2008." *Annals of Indian Academy of Neurology.* 16 July 2013

Morris M, Evans DA, Tangney CC, Bienias JL, and Wilson RS. "Fish Consumption and Cognitive Decline With Age in a Large Community Study." *Arch Neurol* 62.12 (2005): 1849-1853.

Morris MC. "The Role of Nutrition in Alzheimer's Disease: Epidemiological Evidence." *Eur J Neurol* 2009 Sep: 16(Suppl 1) 1-7.

Morris MC, Evans DA, Tangney CC, Bienias JL, and Wilson RS. "Associations of Vegetable and Fruit Consumption With Age-Related Cognitive Change." *Neurology.* 2006;67(8):1370–1376.

Office of the Assistant Secretary for Planning and Evaluation. "National Plan to Address Alzheimer's Disease: 2014 Update." 14 June 2013. *U.S. Department of Health and Human Services.* 23 September 2015 http://aspe.hhs.gov/national-plan-address-alzheimer%E2%80%99s-disease-2014-update.

Qin B, Panickar K, and Anderson R. "Cinnamon: Potential Role in the Prevention of Insulin Resistance, Metabolic Syndrome, and Type 2 Diabetes." *Journal of Diabetes Science and Technology* 4.3 (2010): 685-693.

Quinn JF, et al. "Docosahexaenoic Acid Supplementation and Cognitive Decline in Alzheimer Disease: A Randomized Trial." *JAMA* 304.17 (2010): 1903-1911.

Reger MA, Henderson ST, Hale C, Cholerton B, Baker LD, Watson GS, et al. "Effects of Beta-Hydroxybutyrate on Cognition in Memory-Impaired Adults." *Neurobiol Aging* 25:3 (2004): 311-314.

Ringman JM., et al. "A Potential Role of the Curry Spice Curcumin in Alzheimer's Disease." *Current Alzheimer Research* 2.2 (2005): 131-136.

Roberts, RO., et al. "Relative Intake of Macronutrients Impacts Risk of Mild Cognitive Impairment or Dementia." *Journal of Alzheimer's Disease* 32.2 (2012): 329–339.

Rossi L, Mazzitelli S, Arciello M, Capo CR, and Rotillo G. "Benefits From Dietary Polyphenols for Brain Aging and Alzheimer's Disease." *Neurochemical Research* 33.12 (2008): 2390-2400.

Scarmeas N, et al. "Mediterranean Diet and Mild Cognitive Impairment." *Archives of Neurology* 66.2 (2009): 216-225.

Scarmeas N, et al. "Physical Activity, Diet, and Risk of Alzheimer Disease." *JAMA* 302.6 (2009): 627-637.

Shukitt-Hale B, Lau FC, Joseph JA. "Berry Fruit Supplementation and the Aging Brain." *Journal of Agricultural and Food Chemistry* 56.3 (2008): 636-641.

Sinn N, Milte CM, Street SJ, Buckley JD, Coates AM, Petkov J, and Howe PR. "Effects of N-3 Fatty Acids, EPA V, DHA, on Depressive Symptoms, Quality of Life, Memory, and Executive Function in Older Adults With Mild Cognitive Impairment: A 6-Month Randomised Controlled Trial." 20 September 2011. *PubMed.* 16 July 2013

Smith AD, Smith SM, de Jager CA, Whitbread P, Johnston C, Agacinski G, et al. "Homocysteine-Lowering by B Vitamins Slows the Rate of Accelerated Brain Atrophy in Mild Cognitive Impairment: A Randomized Controlled Trial." *PLoS ONE* 5.9 (2010).

Solfrizzi V, Panza F, Frisardi V, Seripa D, Logroscino G, Imbimbo BP, and Pilotto A. "Diet and Alzheimer's Disease Risk Factors or Prevention: The Current Evidence." *Expert Review of Neurotherapeutics* 11.5 (2011): 677-708.

Taha AY, Henderson ST, and Burnham WM. "Dietary Enrichment With Medium-Chain Triglycerides (AC-1203) Elevates Polyunsaturated Fatty Acids in the Parietal Cortex of Aged Dogs: Implications for Treating Age-Related Cognitive Decline." *Neurochem Res* 34:9 (2009) 1619-1625.

Xu W, Qiu C, Winblad B, and Fratiglioni L. "The Effect of Borderline Diabetes on the Risk of Dementia and Alzheimer's Disease." *Diabetes*
56.1 (2007): 211-216.

Yang F, Lim GP, Begum AN, Ubeda OJ, Simmons MR, Ambegaokar SS,
Chen PP, Kayed R, Glabe CG, Frautschy SA, and Cole GM. "Curcumin
Inhibits Formation of Amyloid Beta Oligomers and Fibrils, Binds
Plaques, and Reduces Amyloid In Vivo." *The Journal of Biological Chem-
istry* 280.7 (2005): 5892-5901.

Index

About Francie Healey

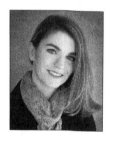

Francie Healey has a Master's Degree in Counseling and is both a Certified Health Counselor and Licensed Mental Health Counselor in private practice in Santa Fe, N.M.

Francie is a health and wellness expert who uses a holistic framework to educate people about what and how to eat in order to feel energized, grounded, and well-nourished. She counsels and educates her clients about holistic nutrition, health and wellness, meal planning, how to cook simple, nutritious meals, food label literacy, developing a healthy relationship with food, achieving and sustaining a healthy weight, emotional eating, reducing cravings, and the connection between food and mood.

In addition to providing health and nutrition counseling, life coaching, and phone consultations, Francie teaches and writes on a variety of health and wellness topics. She wrote and developed recipes for "Protein Power," a cooking feature published in Mothering magazine.

Over the years, Francie has continued to explore the relationship between brain health and nutrition by following new research in the field. Evidence strongly suggests that the progression of Alzheimer's and other forms of cognitive decline can be delayed and in some cases prevented with dietary changes.

Francie says of her practice: "I help my clients to identify the core values in their lives and to understand how emotional eating can affect the realization of their goals. In addition, I help them develop strategies around food that support their vision for wellness in a meaningful and sustainable way."